Cycling improve your sex life?
Herbs keep you stress-free?
Aromatherapy relieve hot flashes?
Tea increase the risk of osteoporosis?

FIND OUT IN

NATURAL CHOICES
FOR MENOPAUSE

NATURAL CHOICES for MENOPAUSE

Marilyn Glenville, Ph.D.

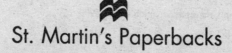

St. Martin's Paperbacks

To all women
whose suffering, confusion, and search for lasting health
and happiness have caused this book to be written

Previously published in the United Kingdom by Kyle Cathie Limited as *Natural Alternatives to HRT*.

NATURAL CHOICES FOR MENOPAUSE

Copyright © 1997 by Marilyn Glenville.
Illustrations © 1997 by Christopher King.

ISBN: 0-312-97013-7

Printed in the United States of America

St. Martin's Paperbacks edition / April 1999

10 9 8 7 6 5 4 3 2 1

A Note To Readers

This book is for informational purposes only and should not be used as a substitute for professional medical advice or care. **Readers are advised to consult a doctor before acting on any of the medical information in this book.**

Contents

Acknowledgments

This book would not have been possible without the help and support of my family, friends, and associates.

In particular I would like to thank Maggie Drummond for the time we spent together and for her help in making this book coherent and readable. Thanks go, too, to Linda McVan, my practice manager, for keeping my practice running smoothly while the writing took place, and to Tammy Mitchum, my practice assistant, who contributed invaluably to the chapter on meals.

My thanks and appreciation are also extended to all my patients and to all the women who have attended my seminars and workshops over the years. Their feedback, humor, and willingness to try a different approach have allowed me to grow and learn from them. Their constant desire to know more about themselves and to take control of their own health inspired me to write this book.

My gratitude also goes to my husband, Kriss, and my children, Matthew, Leonard, and Chantell—their love and support created an environment that enabled this book to become a reality.

I would like to thank Dr. Penny Stanway for reviewing the draft of this book and for her insightful comments—especially her comments on the food allergy section. My thanks also to Kate Oldfield, my editor at Kyle Cathie, for her positive attitude, and to Kyle and her team for their belief in and support for the whole project. Thanks also to Teresa Hale of the Hale Clinic and Dr. Mehta of the Nutri Centre.

My thanks are also due to Gilly Vincent and Jenny Chapman of MultiMedia, who gave much support and encouragement in the early stages of this project, and to Mary Atkinson, who has worked with me many times in the past.

Last, but by no means least, I am indebted to those dedicated medical practitioners, scientists, and nutritional therapists who, sometimes at great personal cost, have worked against the prevailing dogma and so-called conventional "wisdom" to investigate and verify the effectiveness of nutrition in areas that could otherwise have been dominated by drug intervention.

		Supplements	Herbs
MENOPAUSE SELF-HELP GUIDE	Hot flashes	Vitamins E and C and a multivitamin. Minerals: magnesium, calcium and chromium. Bioflavonoids.	Vitex, yarrow, sage, hops, wild yam, dandelion, dong quai.
	Mood swings	Vitamins B complex, E, and beta-carotene. Minerals: magnesium and zinc. Bioflavonoids.	Bach flower remedies, hawthorn, valerian, damiana, St. John's wort.
	Insomnia	Vitamins B complex, C, and E. Minerals: calcium and magnesium. Bioflavonoids.	Passionflower, chamomile, hops, valerian.
	Heavy bleeding	Vitamins A and C. Mineral: iron. Bioflavonoids.	Wild yam, black cohosh, vitex.
	Vaginal dryness	Vitamin E capsule inserted in the vagina.	Calendula cream.
	Osteo-porosis	Vitamin D. Minerals: boron, magnesium, and calcium.	Nettle tea, boneset leaf, marshmallow root, angelica herb.
	Heart disease	Vitamins C and E and beta-carotene. Essential fatty acids.	*Ginkgo biloba*, hawthorn, garlic, ginger.

Diet	Activity
Eat soy foods that contain phyto-estrogens. Drink plenty of mineral water. Avoid spicy foods, caffeine, sugar, alcohol, and refined foods.	Regular aerobic exercise (walking and swimming). Meditation and yoga for relaxation. Essential oils for the bath: geranium, chamomile, jasmine, ylang-ylang.
Eat vegetable oil, nuts, and seeds. Avoid caffeine, sugar, alcohol, and refined foods.	Meditation and yoga to relax the nervous system. Essential oils for the bath: chamomile, juniper, basil, ylang-ylang, geranium.
Drink chamomile tea. Avoid caffeine in any drinks. Eat little and often.	Walking in the fresh air. Yoga and meditation to still the mind. Relaxation technique to be used in bed. Warm bath with aromatherapy oils before going to bed: lavender, geranium, marjoram.
Avoid red meat, excess dairy products, and coffee.	
Drink plenty of mineral water. Eat linseeds, nuts, seeds, and oily fish.	Sexual intercourse and orgasm stimulate blood circulation and lubrication. Pelvic exercises increase blood circulation to the pelvic region.
Eat dark, leafy vegetables, sesame seeds, whole grains. Reduce protein intake and avoid caffeine.	Regular weight-bearing exercise including brisk walking, yoga.
Avoid saturated fat in the form of dairy products and meat. Eat a variety of fruits, vegetables, whole grains, nuts, and seeds.	Regular aerobic exercise. Yoga, meditation, t'ai chi to relax the mind and body.

Foreword

In the United States a large proportion of women take Hormone Replacement Therapy (HRT). This is in contrast with Britain, where women are more cautious and doctors more conservative. There are, however, a number of prominent medical practitioners who are enthusiasts of HRT. One British gynecologist, for example, suggests that *all* women after the menopause should take supplementary hormones. There are also several high-profile organizations that are strong proponents of HRT, as well as some well-known celebrities who like to let the media know they are on HRT.

This book is not meant to tar every doctor with the same brush, and there are many women who are receiving sound medical advice regarding the menopause from their medical practitioners. However, the women I see, almost without exception, have not been happy with the recommendations given to them. There are many doctors now who are aware of the importance of nutrition in a person's health, who adopt a caring, sympathetic approach to the menopause, and who treat it as a natural stage in a woman's life.

It is my hope that those doctors who routinely recommend HRT and consider the menopause an illness will be made aware of the facts contained in this book—facts that may not have been brought to their attention before. I hope that I have presented the facts here in such a way that patients and doctors alike will consider that there may be a more natural, safe, and effective way to care for women's health.

Introduction

The menopause is *not* an illness

This book is all about choices. Choices you didn't know you had. Choices to prevent and treat menopausal symptoms naturally without resorting to Hormone Replacement Therapy (HRT). Because of the nature of my work, I have seen hundreds of women over the years who have been to their family doctor or gynecologist to complain of menopausal symptoms. Their doctor may tell them it's ''their hormones,'' and the only treatment they are offered or told is available is HRT. But many women have the feeling that there must be other possibilities. And indeed there are. Lots of them. The information about these alternatives too often remains stuck in the academic world of scientific research. It is now time that this information is made available to all women. This book is designed to give you the possibility of making an informed choice about your health, enabling you to take responsibility for it at this stage in your life.

As a nutritional therapist I have long believed that diet—what we eat and what we don't eat—is one of the most crucial factors in our health. We are all far too used to receiving negative messages—don't eat this, that, or the other thing. The approach of this book, on the other hand, is positive. I believe that food is the most powerful natural preventative we have, but it is all too often presented to us negatively. My professional experience of helping hundreds of women over the years tells me that menopausal symptoms, and indeed a wide range of other illnesses and disorders, can be prevented and alleviated by adjusting what we eat and making sure we have the necessary nutrients for

1

optimum health. This approach is supported by a mass of scientific research indicating that diet and nutrition are crucial factors in avoiding ill health. But while the scientists are on the hunt for a pharmaceutical "magic bullet," important knowledge about the ability of certain food and nutrients to promote health and well-being remains inaccessible to many women.

This book aims to help you put that knowledge to practical use in your daily life. I believe this positive approach is the key to a smooth passage through the menopause.

This book takes the view that the menopause is a natural stage of a woman's life. As natural and inevitable as the transition from childhood to puberty. Something that our bodies can cope with perfectly well if they are given the chance. This is, of course, in sharp contrast to the view of many medical practitioners who regard the menopause as an illness caused by falling levels of hormones. We are therefore seen as suffering from a hormone deficiency disease. If we are supplied with the hormones in the form of HRT, this deficiency can be corrected and we are "cured."

This argument is often supported by the supposed similarity between the menopause and diabetes. When our own insulin levels are not sufficient to maintain normal blood sugar levels, insulin is supplied from outside and the balance is corrected.

The difference between the menopause and diabetes is that diabetes is not a natural event in our lives. It is not assumed that all of us will get diabetes, but as night follows day all women will pass through the menopause. Diabetes *is* an illness. The menopause *is not*.

Would nature design us as women to reach the menopause and then spend the rest of our lives burdened with myriad uncomfortable symptoms? Maybe we should ask ourselves if the problems many women face at the menopause are not due to nature but to ourselves and our lifestyles.

Moreover, women in many other cultures do not experience the menopause as a crisis demanding medical intervention. Many of them simply do not suffer the physical and emotional symptoms that we in the West are programmed to accept as inevitable. As you will see, this gives us vital clues about the importance of diet and lifestyle and how they have the ability to change our experience of the menopause for the better without our having to take powerful and potentially risky drugs.

In the fall, natural chemical changes occur in a tree and the leaves fall off. Tree surgeons do not attempt to stick the leaves back on, as if this were a symptom of disease, nor do they try to reverse the changes to take the tree back to its level of growth in the summer months. They recognize this stage in the tree's life cycle as natural and accept that during the fall the tree does not need to be covered in leaves. It continues on its natural cycle and blossoms again. And so it is as you pass through the menopause to enjoy the freedom it can bring.

Yes, some women will pass through the menopause smoothly and symptom-free while others will suffer a range of symptoms including hot flashes, night sweats, vaginal dryness, lack of concentration, and depression.

The question to ask is what is causing these symptoms? What can be done to help your body make this transition naturally, efficiently, and comfortably? Nature takes her time; she does things gradually. The change of life is a gradual process, allowing our bodies to get used to the changes and to adapt accordingly. Diet, nutrition, and a healthy lifestyle are crucial to enable your body to do this. In fact many problems experienced by women at the time of the menopause have more to do with poor nutrition than with falling hormone levels. By fundamentally improving your health and using natural remedies where appropriate, you can help your body to balance itself and so be able either to avoid or to treat these symptoms.

This book gives you the information to help yourself through the inevitable change of life in the most positive way, helping you not only to prevent symptoms occurring in the first place, but also to cope with problems if they do arise. It will explain the wealth of natural remedies that are available to you. And, hopefully, by demonstrating that your health can be under your own control, it will inspire you to regard the menopause with optimism.

In our society the focus of the menopause is on loss. We are programmed to dwell on loss—the loss of periods, the loss of the ability to create life, the loss of hormones, the problems of the "empty-nest" syndrome in which the children have grown up and left home. This in itself can bring on depression and other emotional symptoms because the roles that we used to perform are not needed anymore. Some of us can experience an identity crisis.

We could, however, focus on the gains. We gain freedom from the worry of contraception and mental and physical freedom. We have time to pursue our own interests in a serious way. We may want to take up new activities and hobbies or retrain for a new career. If you feel fit and well, the new freedom gives you the opportunity to really concentrate on the things you want to do for yourself. A lady in her fifties whom I've been seeing has decided to buy a motorbike. Margaret Mead, the famous anthropologist, called this feeling of energy and renewal "post-menopausal zest," and it is within the grasp of every woman.

In other societies, this time in a woman's life is seen as one of great wisdom. A time when the emphasis shifts away from doing the chores or working in the fields to the role of lawmaker and counselor to younger couples, when maturity and experience make a significant contribution to the family and society.

Using the information in this book, you can open up your life to the possibilities of good health right through the menopause, approaching the future years with a sense of choice, control, and freedom.

CHAPTER 1

What is the menopause?

The word "menopause," medically speaking, refers to the end of menstruation—the time of your last period. Doctors talk about the "climacteric," medical jargon for the transition period, which may span fifteen to twenty years before, during, and after the menopause. But to most women this transition period is called the "menopause" or the "change."

At the menopause a woman still produces estrogen, but not enough to prepare her womb for pregnancy. Her levels of progesterone fall dramatically and in some cases to zero. Contrary to popular opinion, the menopausal ovary is not a dead or dying organ. It continues to produce estrogen, although in smaller quantities, for at least twelve years after the start of the menopause. And the adrenal glands which sit on top of the kidneys begin to form a type of female hormone which is used alongside the body's diminishing estrogen. Body fat is also a manufacturing plant for estrogen. Fat produces estrogen all our lives—which is why low- or no-fat diets, so often recommended for dieters, are a big mistake for women.

How and why does the menopause happen?

Your monthly cycle is governed by a number of reproductive hormones, the main ones being estrogen, progesterone, follicle stimulating hormone (FSH), and luteinizing hormone (LH). Hormones are chemical messengers, and the word comes from the Greek, meaning "urging on." Carried in the bloodstream, they initiate activity in different organs and body parts; the reproductive hormones control the monthly cycle and help to maintain pregnancy.

At the beginning of each menstrual cycle, the estrogen and progesterone levels are low, and the follicle stimulating hormone (FSH) is secreted from the pituitary gland in the brain which controls the whole of our endocrine (hormone) system.

This begins the process of ovulation by stimulating the ovaries to produce the estrogen hormones. (Estrogen is not one hormone but several grouped together, but for clarity I will use the term "estrogen" to include all of them.) Estrogen is the key hormone responsible for the transition from childhood to womanhood. It causes the breasts to develop and produces our characteristic feminine shape. It also causes the lining of the womb (uterus) to start to thicken each month in anticipation of receiving a fertilized egg.

The estrogen level continues to rise until it reaches a point where the pituitary gland secretes the luteinizing hormone (LH) which triggers ovulation, around the middle of the month. The egg (ovum) is released from a follicle in the ovary at ovulation and passes down the Fallopian tube.

After ovulation, the ovaries then secrete progesterone, which prevents any further ovulation from taking place in that cycle. If fertilization does not occur, the lining of the womb breaks down and you get a period. At the same time there is a dramatic and rapid fall in the levels of estrogen and progesterone, and with this drop in hormone levels, the cycle then starts all over again. If fertilization does occur, the ovum implants itself into the thick and nourishing wall of the womb, where it begins to develop.

Symptoms associated with the menopause, such as hot flashes, night sweats, etc., can all start well before your periods stop. Ovulation becomes less likely because estrogen levels decline during the first two weeks of the cycle, which means that progesterone will not be produced in the second half. But the body has already experienced other changes. We start off with a certain number of egg cells from birth. As they are used up and die off over the years, only a few egg cells remain by the time of the menopause.

Without the rising levels of estrogen in the first two weeks to send a message back to the ovaries to produce smaller amounts of FSH, the levels of FSH in the blood-stream keep rising. So a period can still happen without ovulation occurring but with rising levels of FSH and LH. A simple blood test can be done which measures the level of FSH. If it is high, it shows that it is likely that you are menopausal.

There are three distinct phases of the menopause:

1. Pre-menopause—periods are still regular, but the first symptoms, such as hot flashes and mood changes, may appear.
2. Peri-menopause—the function of the ovaries declines, the periods can become irregular, and symptoms may be more severe.
3. Post-menopause—this is from the last period onward. Of course, we can only know it is the last period after twelve months with no periods. Some women can go six months without a period, and then another one arrives. Once a year has passed with no periods, it can be said that you are post-menopausal.

Your hormones affect you mentally and physically. They have an impact on breast tissue, body hair, and the physical shape that distinguishes you as a woman. They are also closely connected with your emotional and psychological well-being, as any woman who has suffered from pre-menstrual syndrome will testify. As the hormones change during the monthly cycle, so does the way you think, in terms of your confidence and self-esteem: the way you view yourself and the world.

Nature has designed your hormones to work in harmony, each one dependent on the other and operating as a whole system. When your hormones are in proper balance, you feel emotionally and physically well. Exactly the same principle holds true for the years leading up to the menopause. The level of your hormones is changing, but when you are in good health they are changing in exactly the way they should. The menopause is not a deficiency disease.

When will the menopause happen?

The average age for the onset of the menopause in the United Kingdom is fifty-one. But perfectly normal women may have a much earlier menopause, with their periods stopping before the age of forty-five, while others find they carry on menstruating till their mid fifties.

A premature menopause, one that happens before the age of forty, can be caused by a number of factors. It can happen spontaneously when the supply of egg cells in the ovaries becomes exhausted. It can also be induced artificially by radiation or removal of the ovaries. If you are advised to have a hysterectomy, find out whether your ovaries are also going to be removed. If they are, ask why. Some doctors may tell you it is done as a prevention against ovarian cancer. The thinking is that if you don't have your womb, you won't need your ovaries. But beware. If your ovaries are removed, you will go into a surgical menopause, and this can be traumatic for you and your body. As it is a sudden event, the female hormone supply from the ovaries will be cut off overnight, whereas going through a natural menopause (even without a womb) can take anywhere from fifteen to twenty years as the hormone levels gradually decline. Nature takes things gradually, so that your body can adjust to the changes at its own pace, and then the menopause can be just a smooth change in your life. If you are not of menopausal age and you have your ovaries removed, this is one of the situations in which HRT may be necessary.

The timing of the average menopause is linked to a number of factors:

❑ The timing of your mother's menopause is a good indication of your own. But even if you know she had a difficult menopause, there is no reason to fear that you will suffer in the same way. You will see later that there are plenty of things you can do to improve your own health.

❑ Smokers will tend to have an earlier menopause by about two years. It seems that smoking has an effect on the secretion of estrogens from the ovaries, causing a decrease in these hormone levels. This can also be seen in infertile women of childbearing age who are smokers. Their hormone patterns begin to mimic those of a menopausal woman.

❑ Women who suffer from PMS tend to have a later menopause by about a year.

❑ A hysterectomy, without the removal of the ovaries, can accelerate the onset of the menopause by about five years.

❑ Women who have fibroids may experience a later menopause because they have higher levels of estrogen.

❑ Women who weigh more than 140 pounds (63.5kg.) can have a later menopause because of the estrogen manufactured in the fat cells.

❑ Poor nutrition can bring on an earlier menopause.

❑ Women who have not had children tend to have an earlier menopause.

It would seem more beneficial to have a later menopause because of the protective effects of the female hormones for bone health. But a woman who is still menstruating around the age of fifty-five should have a check-up in case there is a medical reason, such as fibroids, for the continuing periods.

How do the hormones estrogen and progesterone affect you?

You may find it surprising to know that a woman's body converts her main sex hormones, estrogen and progesterone, from cholesterol. So the hormones are inextricably linked and have the same "starting block"—cholesterol—although they have different functions.

ESTROGEN'S ROLE

❑ At puberty, estrogen is responsible for our female shape, including the growth and development of our breasts and the growth of pubic and underarm hair.
❑ Estrogen causes the womb lining to thicken in the first half of the menstrual cycle.
❑ Estrogen softens the cervix and produces the right quality of vaginal secretions to allow the sperm to swim and to lubricate us during intercourse.
❑ Estrogen maintains the health and functioning of our genital organs.
❑ This hormone has a stimulating effect on both the womb and breasts in terms of cell growth.
❑ Estrogen lifts our mood and gives us a feeling of well-being.

PROGESTERONE'S ROLE

❑ Progesterone helps to maintain pregnancy.
❑ It protects us against the "building" effects of estrogen, which are linked to the development of breast and womb cancer.
❑ Progesterone prevents further ovulation from taking place in the second half of the menstrual cycle, closes the cervix at that time, and produces a thick mucus, hostile to sperm, which prevents its passage into the womb.

As these two hormones decline during the menopause, the pattern of our periods change. The periods may

1. Stop abruptly. After having regular periods for many years, you may find you just stop menstruating without any warning.
2. The number of days you bleed in each cycle becomes shorter and shorter, and the blood flow may also diminish, but the periods are still regular.
3. The periods may become very irregular. Some can become heavier with large gaps in between.

4. Most women find they get less bleeding less often, but there are plenty of variations. It is the change from your normal pattern that is the main indicator of the menopause.

Nature takes her time, she does things gradually. The change of life is a gradual process, allowing your body to get used to the changes and to adapt accordingly. If your body is healthy, these changes can happen smoothly and comfortably. The hormone systems in your body are interlinked and work in harmony with each other. But modern gynecology looks at just the symptoms of the menopause and tries to correct those instead of looking at our bodies as whole integrated systems. When a woman goes through the menopause, modern medicine may prescribe her estrogen because the level of that hormone is falling. But that is not the only thing that is happening. What about the progesterone, which has stopped altogether? What about the FSH level, which is soaring? What about all the other subtle changes in hormone balance which cannot even be measured or that we don't even know about? As one thing changes, so does everything else; this is how nature works. Just as we drop a stone into a pond and the ripples are seen far away, so, too, if we interfere with the balance of hormones, the body will try to compensate and the effects can be noticeable as a different imbalance. This is the single biggest reason why women should think twice—and a few more times—before taking Hormone Replacement Therapy. The real question to ask is what is causing you to feel these symptoms? What can be done to help your body go through this transition naturally, efficiently, and comfortably? By increasing your health and using natural remedies where appropriate, you can help your body to balance itself.

CHAPTER 2

What are the symptoms of the menopause?

The list of problems widely believed to be associated with the menopause makes lengthy and frightening reading. It really makes you wonder if there has been a fear campaign from interested parties to encourage women to take HRT. As you can see, the list includes life-threatening problems like osteoporosis, as well as psychological disorders:

- hot flashes,
- night sweats,
- irritability,
- declining libido,
- osteoporosis,
- weight gain,
- vaginal dryness,
- aging skin,
- changes in hair quality,
- headaches,
- mood swings, including depression,
- lack of energy,
- joint pains.

The truth is that many of these so-called "menopausal symptoms" may have little to do with the menopause. Some are just a natural part of the aging process and affect middle-aged men just as much as they affect women. Others may be related to particular events in our lives that have nothing to with our hormones. The classic example of this is the "empty-nest" syndrome which many women have to face up to in their late forties or early fifties when children leave home. This can be quite a crisis. You carry on worrying about your children, but you may no longer have daily contact with them. To try to explain away these powerful and legitimate feelings in terms of falling hormone levels is to dismiss many women's important experience of motherhood. At this time in their lives, many women are trying to cope with elderly parents too. It can be very stressful, far more stressful than looking after any number of young children. Few things are more depressing than having to watch a much-loved parent in the final stages of illness. It is quite wrong to blame all these emotional problems on the menopause. When you analyze it, there are only a few symptoms that can be truly called menopausal. This is not to say that these symptoms are trivial. Some women suffer severely from them. Others sail through the menopause without any problems at all.

Hot flashes

Many women will have hot flashes and night sweats at around the time of the menopause. Hot flashes can start as a feeling of heat in the face, neck, or body and the heat can spread up or down. These can be experienced in different ways. Women may have no outward signs of redness or sweating, or may sweat profusely and become extremely red in the face. Some women may react with palpitations; others just experience a general feeling of increased body heat, as if somebody had raised their body temperature. Equally some women find the hot flashes very uncomfortable, while others may just find them inconvenient.

No one really knows what causes the hot flashes. One theory suggests that they are triggered by falling levels of estrogen. Another theory considers that it is the higher levels of FSH that are the trigger. Hot flashes are termed "vasomotor" symptoms, because the size of the blood vessels changes as part of the body's temperature-control system. Blood vessels dilate—that is, get larger—to allow more blood through the vessels in order to cool us down. It is that automatic mechanism, for instance, that makes us sweat on a hot day. After a flash, many women feel cold and shivery, and after taking off layers of clothes, want to put them back on again. These flashes can occur many times during the day and last from just a few seconds to thirty minutes. At night, the flashes are called night sweats, and a woman may wake up to find herself drenched in sweat and need to dry herself and change her nightgown. Since the night sweats are constantly waking her up, her pattern of sleep becomes disturbed, resulting in tiredness, depression, and irritability. Most of us would feel like this if we were woken up a number of times each night!

Vaginal changes

As the level of estrogen falls, the walls of the vagina become thinner, and the blood flow to this area is restricted, causing a lack of lubrication. Doctors describe this as vaginal atrophy, which actually means wasting away, becoming useless. It's a nasty term, guaranteed to make any woman feel she is about to become a dried-up husk. In fact, it's a real case of "use it or lose it."

Although the vagina does not expand so much, it is still quite large enough to accommodate an erect penis. But the thinning of the vagina can encourage bacterial infections such as cystitis. Staying sexually active is a must. Regular sex or masturbation stimulates the blood flow into the vaginal area, reducing dryness. The muscle contractions during orgasm promote the health of the vagina.

Your waterworks are also affected by vaginal changes. The lining walls of the bladder and urethra (the tube linking the bladder to the outside) shrink and become thinner and drier and can become more liable to infection if they crack and split. You may feel the need to urinate more frequently, or find you leak a bit when you sneeze, cough, or laugh. The good news is that there are plenty of natural ways to deal with these symptoms.

Psychological changes

Our hormones certainly have a powerful impact on the way we feel. Anyone who has suffered premenstrual tension, and that includes most women at one time or another, don't need to be told that. In fact the list of so-called "menopausal" symptoms bears a remarkable similarity to those associated with PMS.

• lack of self-esteem,
• less energy and motivation,
• lack of self-confidence,
• mood swings,
• irritability,
• forgetfulness,
• depression,
• anxiety,
• feeling of losing control,
• feeling unable to cope,
• loss of sex drive,
• feeling close to tears,
• vulnerability,
• lack of concentration.

These symptoms can be due to a hormonal imbalance, which can be experienced by women at any point in their lives from the time they have their first period. They can also be due to stress, for example, as both men and women can suffer equally from them. There is nothing specifically "menopausal" about them at all. It reminds me of one patient who had suffered several of these symptoms quite severely all her life. When she was young, she was told that everything would be all right once she had babies. After that she was told that things would sort themselves out once she had the menopause . . .

Women who suffer from PMS can find their symptoms getting much worse at the time of the menopause. Others, who have not had PMS, may suddenly find they have some of these symptoms. Some of the emotional changes may simply be due to broken sleep caused by night sweats. Experiencing even a few of these would be enough to turn most of us into a caricature of an emotional woman, driving her family mad with depression and mood swings. There is, of course, an entire industry devoted to convincing middle-aged women that they are suffering from the menopause—and that taking HRT to "top up" their hormones is the best solution to the problem. Middle-aged women suffering these symptoms may also be prescribed antidepressants and tranquilizers by their doctors, which are rarely beneficial. Most of these drugs are potentially addictive. The correct way to look at these psychological symptoms is as a continuum of hormonal imbalance, not as something directly caused by the menopause. And the correct way to cope with them is to restore the proper balance of mind as well as body through the natural measures outlined in this book.

CHAPTER 3

What is Hormone Replacement Therapy (HRT)?

HRT has been seen as a universal panacea, a solution to all menopausal problems from aging skin to osteoporosis. It has been pushed by the media and is supposed to give us the energy of a spring chicken and the libido of a teenager. The principle behind HRT is that it supplies us with hormones when our own production slows down. Thus we can avoid the hot flashes, the night sweats, and many of the other "symptoms" of the menopause with the medical equivalent of one-stop shopping. Dr. Ellen Grant, who wrote *The Bitter Pill*, suggests that HRT, which delivers a constant level of estrogen, is like having a car stuck in a single gear. Surely it is better to let our own pituitary gland and ovaries work together to make fine adjustments constantly for our hormone needs at each moment, like a car with automatic gears? Given optimum health, our hormones are able to balance themselves. Our bodies are able to make the judgment on whether we have too much of one hormone or need to produce more of another: just like a furnace thermostat, which will turn on the heat if the room temperature drops and turn it off again when the room heats up.

Estrogen therapy has been around since the 1930s, when injections of estrogen were given for menopausal symptoms. Because of the inconvenience of this form of treatment, implant pellets of estrogen were introduced in 1938. HRT was originally called Estrogen Replacement Therapy, because only estrogen was given as the treatment. However, it became clear that giving estrogen alone could increase the risk of cancer of the womb and breasts.[1] When research

17

studies appeared to demonstrate that this increased risk could be up to seven times higher for womb cancer, there was panic.[2] Estrogen therapy declined sharply in popularity. Then progestogen, the synthetic version of progesterone, was added to the therapy for ten to fourteen days each month, and HRT, using both hormone drugs, was re-marketed. Since then, there seems to be no end to what HRT can do for us. There is always something new. Over the last year, I have seen newspaper reports that HRT might help patients with inflammatory bowel disease, postnatal depression, premenstrual migraine—and prevent Alzheimer's disease. An opera singer found that it had a wonderful effect on her voice. Most of us are much more interested in just what the risks of HRT really are. The main reasons for the addition of progestogen to HRT are to protect the womb lining from over-stimulation and subsequent cancer and to cause a regular bleed. Women who have had a hysterectomy obviously cannot get womb cancer, so they are not given progestogen.

It is important to make clear the difference between progesterone (our own naturally occurring hormone) and progestogen (the synthetic hormone in the Pill and HRT). Many people, even doctors, treat them as the same thing, and they are not. Progesterone is made just prior to ovulation by the corpus luteum and is the major female hormone for the second half of the menstrual cycle. It is absolutely necessary to maintain a pregnancy. As progesterone rises at ovulation our body temperature rises, ready to "incubate" the fertilized egg. If we are pregnant, progesterone continues to rise. If we are not pregnant, both estrogen and progesterone levels fall, and we have a period. If a woman does not produce sufficient progesterone when the egg is fertilized, she can miscarry.

Progestogens, on the other hand, are synthetic. Though they are able to fulfill many of progesterone's functions, the human body has difficulty "recognizing" and coping with progestogens because they are not natural—hence the well-known side effects, such as mood swings, depression, etc. These synthetic progestogens are used for their progesterone-like action, but they can have additional male or female hormone effects. So one type of progestogen may cause enlargement of the breasts, while another can increase the growth of facial hair. All somewhat alarming.

The sex hormones estrogen and progesterone are both steroids. They are closely related to the anabolic steroids which some athletes have used as body builders. HRT contains the same combinations of estrogens and progestogens that make up the Pill. The difference between the Pill and HRT lies in the difference in the estrogens by dose and chemical structure. Most of the combined oral Pills contain ethinyl estradiol, which is a synthetic estrogen, whereas those used in HRT are usually referred to as "natural." "Natural," in this case, means that they have been extracted from pigs' ovaries or pregnant mares' urine, a substance particularly high in estrogen, (hence the name Premarin, one of the best-selling HRTs, and also Prempak C). Not all the estrogens in the mixture are natural to humans, and some can behave like ethinyl estradiol, the synthetic hormone, which tends to affect liver metabolism by producing changes in blood clotting and blood fat levels. The progestogens used in the Pill and HRT are the same, but in HRT the progestogen is given only for ten to twelve days of each cycle. Because of the close similarity between the Pill and HRT, it is not surprising that many of the side effects reported by women—water retention, weight gain, headaches, and depression—are the same.

Some women stopped taking HRT when disturbing reports appeared in the media about its production. In 1995, a representative of the World Society for the Protection of Animals (WSPA) was part of a team that inspected thirty-two farms in Canada, all of which were contracted to supply mare's urine. The following passage is extracted from WSPA's report, *HRT*, published in 1996:

". . . after mares have become pregnant, they are brought into barns and housed in individual stalls. A harness-type device . . . is attached to the animals' rear quarters so that their urine can be collected. The horses spend most of the next six months in these stalls while their estrogen-rich urine is collected.

Often the horses' stalls were too small to allow the animals to lie down comfortably. In nearly all of the farms visited, our inspector saw tethers that were so short that mares were unable to lay their head on the ground. . . . In all but a few farms, water was being restricted . . . it is suspected that this is practiced in order to ensure that urine has a high concentration of oestrogen."

WSPA's findings from the visit were shared by other members of the inspection team, which included an expert from the Royal School of Veterinary Studies in Edinburgh, which also published a report, *Report of Findings During Visit to Pregnant Mare's Urine (PMU) Farms, Saskatchewan 17–19 February, 1995*, in which it described the stalls in most barns as "totally unsuitable for horses . . ."

Since this 1995 inspection, Edinburgh University has reported that

"Wyeth-Ayerst [the company that makes Premarin] has announced that changes have been made at certain farms and that veterinary supervision has been stepped up. However, the company has refused to allow WSPA, as well as local animal welfare inspectors, to re-visit any of the farms . . .

Adult horses are not the only ones to suffer in the production of Premarin. For every pregnant mare . . . a foal is born each year. Most of these young animals are of little value to the farmers. Each year thousands are sold off cheaply and fattened up at giant feed lots before being slaughtered. Many end up on dinner plates in Japan or Europe or are used to make dog food."

Other organizations that are concerned about the treatment of these horses include: PETA (People for the Ethical Treatment of Animals); The Humane Society of the United States; the RSPCA; and the University of Edinburgh's Department of Veterinary Clinical Studies. Both WSPA and PETA have information packs which are available by mail.

Different methods of taking HRT

Hormone Replacement Therapy can now be taken in a variety of different ways. There is a large range of HRT products available, including implants, tablets, skin patches, creams, vaginal pessaries, and gels. They are usually prescribed by your doctor.

IMPLANTS

Subcutaneous HRT is a pellet containing six months' supply of estrogen which is inserted beneath the skin of the lower abdomen. Implants have a number of advantages. Unlike oral HRT, they bypass the liver and go directly into the bloodstream, which means that the dose of hormones can be lower but still just as effective. Many women find implants convenient. Once inserted they can be forgotten about. But unless you have had a hysterectomy, you should still be taking progestogen tablets for some of the time to induce a bleed. And there are also disadvantages. Once inserted, wrong doses cannot easily be changed. It can be difficult to remove an implant if you decide to stop HRT. More worryingly, some women using implants can develop a form of dependency on the hormone, requiring ever larger amounts for the HRT to work effectively. The symptoms associated with the menopause seem to recur at shorter and shorter intervals, so that the implant has to be replaced much more frequently. When their hormone levels are tested, these women often have much higher than normal levels of estrogen, and yet they are still suffering from menopausal symptoms. It may be that they are not absorbing the estrogen properly or that the body becomes "used" to a particular dose and therefore needs ever-increasing amounts to elicit relief of the symptoms. A form of estrogen "addiction" has also been suggested.

TABLETS

The most common way of taking estrogen and progestogen is by mouth. Women who have had a hysterectomy are given only estrogen. The estrogen and progestogen tablets can be prescribed in a number of ways. In the most common pattern estrogen is taken continuously every day, and progestogen is taken from day fourteen to day twenty-five of the cycle. Once the progestogen is stopped, a withdrawal bleed is induced which mimics a period. This is called continuous therapy, because estrogen is taken all the time.

In cyclical therapy estrogen is taken for the first twenty-one days of the cycle, and progestogen is taken from day nine through day twenty-one, so from day twenty-two there are seven days with no medication, and a withdrawal bleed takes place.

For many women, one of the advantages of the menopause is the freedom from periods, so the idea of resuming their periods and perhaps having them into their eighties if they stay on HRT is not appealing. Another approach is to use the hormones in such a way that a bleed occurs only every three months. Estrogen is taken continuously for three months, and progestogen added only at the end of the third month to induce a bleed.

The other choice is a no-bleed HRT called Livial (Tibolone). This is a synthetic compound given continuously, and there is no withdrawal bleed. The prescribing recommendations for this drug specify that it should be given only to those women who have had one complete year free of periods.

SKIN PATCHES

Estrogen is contained under the patch, which is worn on the torso, below the waistline, and the hormone enters the body through the skin. Patches are usually changed every three to four days. Progestogen can be taken in pill form from days fourteen through twenty-five, or a combination skin patch can be used which delivers the progestogen as well as the estrogen. Some women find that the patch irritates their skin.

CREAMS

Estrogen-containing cream is inserted directly into the vagina with an applicator. The creams are usually used for treating vaginal dryness, itchiness, and discomfort. The dose is too low to help with hot flashes.

VAGINAL PESSARIES

The pessaries contain estrogen, which helps with vaginal dryness and pain on passing urine. Again the dose is too low to help with hot flashes.

GELS

Estrogen is available in a gel form, which is rubbed onto the lower abdomen and absorbed through the skin as with a patch. Many women have found that they react to the adhesive in a patch, so the use of a gel may overcome this.

HRT—the side effects

In the United States, doctors use a manual called *The Physician's Desk Reference*. Drug companies are required by law to state the risks of their drugs in this manual. *The Physician's Desk Reference* lists the possible side effects for HRT, which include

- endometrial (womb) cancer,
- undesirable weight gain/loss,
- breast tenderness/enlargement,
- bloating,
- mental depression,
- thrombophlebitis (inflammation of the wall of a vein),
- elevated blood pressure,
- reduced carbohydrate tolerance,

- reduced glucose tolerance,
- skin rashes,
- hair loss,
- abdominal cramps,
- vaginal candidiasis (thrush),
- jaundice,
- nausea,
- vomiting,
- cystitis-like syndrome.

Although research has not shown that women on HRT gain weight—other than the weight gain that would normally be associated with aging—I find that it is one of the greatest concerns of the women who come to see me. Their main complaint is the "sudden" increase in weight (and increases in breast size by up to two cups larger) soon after starting HRT. I also see women not on HRT, and the weight gain is definitely different between the two groups.

So this is a prime symptom that makes women want to stop taking HRT. They are also concerned about psychological changes—feelings of being suicidal, feeling "not there," and headaches. Organizations like the Amarant Trust, the British charity that promotes the use of HRT, have drawn attention to the fact that many British women who try HRT give it up after only a few months. It believes the reason is that women do not persevere for long enough and do not try alternative HRT products, and that their doctors do not spend sufficient time and effort explaining the therapy to them. There are, however, many doctors who have reservations about the over-prescribing of HRT. Many women feel perfectly well on HRT. But it is not surprising that others come to the conclusion that the side effects they experience are worse than the symptoms the HRT is designed to "cure." And as the years roll on, there is increasing evidence that taking HRT involves some serious health risks which many of us would rather avoid.

WOMB CANCER

A study in the *New England Journal of Medicine* in 1975 showed that women using estrogen could have a seven times greater risk of developing endometrial (womb) cancer.[2] This has been confirmed by a number of other studies, and estrogen therapy has also been linked with endometrial hyperplasia—overgrowth of the lining of the womb.[3] Estrogen's role in the body is to increase cell growth, so it is logical that it would directly affect the parts of a woman that are most receptive to estrogen, such as the womb and breasts.

Estrogen and progestogen together (opposed hormone replacement therapy) are now given to women who still have a womb. But the risk of endometrial cancer is still three times the rate of that for women who don't take HRT at all.[4]

In *The Physician's Desk Reference* which lists the side effects of drugs, the makers of one type of estrogen state, "Estrogens have been reported to increase the risk of endometrial carcinoma." In other words, they are in no doubt that the estrogen in HRT is linked to womb cancer.

Unfortunately, researchers from King's College Menopause Clinic in London have found that this increased cell growth in the womb (hyperplasia) does not stop directly when the HRT is abandoned. A report in the *British Medical Journal* in 1990 concluded that progestogens needed to be taken for an additional two years after stopping HRT to keep the womb lining under control.[5]

BREAST CANCER

There was another frightening discovery in 1976, when the highly respected *New England Journal of Medicine* reported a study linking menopausal estrogens to an increase in breast cancer. Numerous studies since then have confirmed this finding, showing that estrogen can increase the risk of breast cancer by up to 60 percent.[6]

Is there any protection, then, for the breasts by combining estrogen and progestogen? The answer seems to be no, and combined HRT may even increase the risk. A landmark study in 1989 of 23,244 women, which was reported in the *New England Journal of Medicine*, found that women using HRT had twice the risk of breast cancer after nine years.[7]

The most worrying finding was that those women who were taking combined estrogen and progestogen had over *four* times the risk of developing breast cancer after six years' use. They concluded from the incidence of breast cancer in those women taking HRT that breast cancer "is not prevented and may even be increased by the addition of progestogens."

An editorial in the same edition of the *New England Journal of Medicine* commented that the findings confirm early results that estrogen plus progestogen could be more carcinogenic (cancer forming) than estrogen alone.[8] However, the comment continued, "The data are not conclusive enough to warrant any immediate change in the way we approach hormone replacement."

By now you should be speechless. But in 1992 the same research team announced that they had followed up these 23,244 women over the intervening four years and found the same risks for breast cancer with estrogen alone that they had found in 1989. However, they also found that the breast cancer risk of taking opposed HRT (estrogen and progestogen) was even greater than they had originally thought.[9]

I have seen women who have been put on HRT to help with menopausal symptoms (such as hot flashes, etc.) and then been told to take Tamoxifen (the anti-estrogen hormone) to help protect them against the risk of breast cancer, which might be caused as a side effect from taking the HRT. Tamoxifen has a list of side effects of its own (noted in the *British National Formulary*, a drug reference book published by the British Medical Association and the Royal Pharmaceutical Society of Great Britain) including rashes, alopecia (hair loss), and visual disturbances. It is possible that these women will later be given more medication to help get rid of the side effects caused by the Tamoxifen (which was, as you remember, given to reduce the side effects of the HRT in the first place). Interestingly, the first side effect mentioned for Tamoxifen in the *British National Formulary* is hot flashes! More HRT needed?

STROKES AND BLOOD CLOTS

Opposed HRT (in which both estrogen and progestogen are used) has a similar effect on the circulatory system and our veins and arteries as does the Pill. It can lead to risks connected with raised blood pressure, migraine, strokes, and thrombosis. You must ask yourself: is taking HRT worth the risk?

HEART DISEASE

Second to osteoporosis, heart disease is the reason given to many women for starting HRT because it supposedly decreases the risk of heart disease (see Chapter 9, page 161 for more details). In fact the Framingham Study (the best-known long-term study of 670 women on HRT in Framingham, Massachusetts), which reported its findings in the *New England Journal of Medicine* in 1985, showed that the risk of heart disease actually increased on taking the hormones.[10] Since HRT contains the same combination of hormones as the Pill (with differences in dose and structure), the *British Medical Journal* in December 1992 stated, "Many doctors have been surprised to discover that a hormonal treatment they had learned to avoid in women at risk of cardiovascular disease is now being specifically advised in this situation." Yet HRT is currently touted as a preventive measure.

OSTEOPOROSIS

One of the other main reasons women take HRT is that they are told that it will protect their bones. Such is the fear of osteoporosis that women have been persuaded that HRT is a prime preventive measure. It is quite extraordinary that women are prepared to take powerful hormones to try to prevent something that may never happen anyway—or that can be avoided in most cases by perfectly benign means such as diet and exercise. It's even more extraordinary when you consider the full meaning of the research into the impact of HRT on bone health. The Framingham Study showed that only women who had taken estrogen for at least seven years had significantly higher bone mineral density than women who had not had estrogen.[11] Even those who had been on estrogen therapy for ten years were not protected from fractures. Their bone mineral density declined rapidly as soon as they stopped taking estrogen. By the time they were seventy-five to eighty years of age—the age at which most fractures happen—their bone mass was only marginally higher than the women of comparable age who had never had estrogen at all. They had only a trivial advantage.

The conclusion is that for HRT to be effective against osteoporosis, women who start taking it at the menopause must take it for decades. In fact, they must take it for the rest of their lives if it is osteoporosis they are worried about. Or perhaps not think about taking it until much later—nearer the time that fractures happen. This is perhaps one sensible option worth exploring—but one which would blow a big hole in the billion-dollar market for HRT products which needs to get women onto HRT as soon as possible. Even worse, the Framingham study was based on women taking estrogen alone, rather than the estrogen-progestogen combination which is now the most widely used form of HRT. The truth is that we really have no idea whether women taking the combined HRT will get any bone benefits at all. Yet every frightening leaflet you pick up about osteoporosis proclaims the efficacy of HRT, while the reality is that very little of any practical relevance has actually been proven. As Dr. Bruce Ettinger, an osteoporosis expert, says, ''It definitely works, but you're talking about taking hormones for ten years—maybe twenty to thirty years—to prevent a largely asymptomatic, self-limited disease. And what are you offering—the risk of endometrial cancer? Lifelong periods? Endometrial biopsies?''[12] HRT is certainly not a ''cure'' for osteoporosis.

MOOD SWINGS

Progestogens can cause profound side effects similar to those associated with premenstrual syndrome (PMS), such as breast tenderness, abdominal cramps, fluid retention, weight gain, headaches, depression, irritability, and tiredness. So not only are women experiencing these side effects, but they are also having a withdrawal bleed when the progestogen is finished for each cycle. Many women are so relieved to have finished with monthly bleeding (it's one of the benefits of the menopause!) that they do not like the idea of having it again. These are some of the reasons women stop using HRT. Doctors have also found that when women realize that it is the progestogens causing the negative aspects of HRT, they may omit those tablets altogether, taking only the estrogen, and so leaving themselves with an increased risk of womb cancer. Only a sixth of the women who start taking Hormone Replacement Therapy continue to take it for a year.

Chris, forty-eight, came to see me with severe depression, constantly crying, not wanting to get out of bed, and even feeling suicidal. She had no history of psychological problems, was socially active, and helped her husband run a successful business. She mentioned that she was taking HRT and had noticed herself that after she had finished taking the progestogen tablets for that cycle she started to feel slightly better and then went downhill again once she had to start taking them. A visit to her doctor had resulted in her being given sleeping tablets plus an antidepressant, as it was obviously "her age." She came off the HRT with medical guidance, has been looking after herself with a recommended program of vitamins and minerals, and is now actively back at work and feeling "interested in life again."

What is extraordinary about this case, and many others like it, is that many members of the medical profession seem unwilling to entertain the notion that it is HRT that may be the problem. Typically the women will be dosed up with something else in addition. This puts them on a treadmill of medication. Your body and mind are so interrelated that any chemicals taken (such as HRT) can have a profound effect on how you look at life. If you took LSD, you would not be surprised to "see" reality differently. In my experience, our physical health is much easier to change than our mental health. When the women I have seen become physically well and hormonally balanced, they feel in control and able to enjoy their lives.

What are the contraindications for HRT?

Contraindications are medical conditions you may have, or be at risk of, that mean you should not take a particular drug or medicine. For HRT these are listed in the *British National Formulary* as:

* liver disease,
* breast cancer,
* history of thrombosis.

Another list of risk factors is given under the heading "Cautions." If you suffer from any of these you should think twice before taking HRT:

* high blood pressure,
* benign (not cancerous) breast disease, e.g. breast cysts,
* fibroids (benign tumors in the womb),
* migraine,
* endometriosis (the lining of the womb growing in other places than just the womb).

HRT has an effect on the whole circulatory system—your blood circulation, your veins, and your arteries. So it can increase the risks of raised blood pressure, migraine, strokes, and thrombosis. It also increases your levels of estrogen, the "building" hormone, and hence the risks of breast tissue changes, fibroids, and endometriosis. And there is the "domino" effect on other vital organs: the liver, for instance, which is your "waste disposal unit" and helps remove excess hormones from the body. If it has to work overtime to remove hormones added into your body from HRT, its function can be affected, increasing the possibility of liver disease.

It is obvious from looking at the evidence that there are risks involved in taking HRT. There are also some women who cannot take it because of their medical or family history. The scientists don't all agree over the percentage of the risks, especially with breast cancer, but they do agree there are increased risks. In a situation like this, it is necessary for us as women to weigh up the positive and negative effects of HRT. For some women who have had a surgical menopause early in life, HRT may be necessary. The sudden fall in hormone levels when their ovaries are removed is a tough challenge for the body. But women going through a natural menopause (with or without a womb) are in a very different situation. Are the benefits of HRT really worth the risks—particularly when there are plenty of natural alternatives for coping with the symptoms of the Change?

CHAPTER 4

"Natural" progesterone—why this is not the answer either

In 1966 Dr. Robert Wilson, a New York gynecologist, wrote a book called *Feminine Forever*, extolling the virtues of estrogen replacement for women at the menopause. By taking it for the rest of our lives, he declared, we could partake forever of the "fountain of youth," as he described it. Dr. Wilson, a charming man, whom I once met, was certainly sincere enough in his desire to help women who experienced difficulties at the menopause. But it was his theories, expounded in this best-selling book, that created the concept of the menopause as a deficiency disease, an illness that could have dire consequences if left untreated. "Women will be emancipated only when the shackles of hormonal deprivation are loosened," burbled the foreword, written by another eminent doctor. The message was that we ignored the prospect of estrogen replacement at our peril. It had a huge impact on popular health thinking at the time. Dr. Wilson got quite carried away by it all, claiming there was ample evidence that the whole course of history has been changed not only by the presence of estrogen but by its absence. Unstable estrogen-starved women, he postulated, were a misery to themselves and everyone else, causing, at the extreme, alcoholism, drug addiction, divorce, and broken homes. As you can imagine, this changed the thinking of many women and doctors for decades. Estrogen replacement became part of mainstream medicine, the great savior. Then disaster struck.

Twenty years later, doctors found that cases of endometrial cancer had risen greatly (to between four and eight times higher than that in non-hormone users) among the

early generation of estrogen takers. Progestogens were then
added to help balance out the side effects of the estrogen,
so that "estrogen replacement therapy" became "hormone
replacement therapy" and most women were required to
take both the hormones, as explained in the previous chapter. Everyone became a little more cautious about hailing
estrogen as the best thing since sliced bread.

All this happened decades ago. But we are now today
seeing a similar pattern developing over another hormone:
progesterone—or natural progesterone, as its growing number of fans prefer to describe it. Enter the new hyped-up
wonder hormone, now hailed as the real and "natural" hormone replacement. Is history merely repeating itself? Are
we now going through another phase in which everyone is
jumping on the bandwagon by promoting progesterone as
safe and effective before the true picture has been established?

According to its supporters, progesterone can help bone
density and "cure" an amazing selection of menopausal
symptoms. Here is a list of some of them:

- anxiety,
- black circles under the eyes,
- blurred vision,
- breast pain and problems,
- cold hands and feet,
- constipation,
- cyclic acne,
- depression,
- disturbances in appetite,
- dry skin,
- exhaustion,
- fibroids,
- infertility,
- insomnia,
- irritability,
- lack of sex drive,
- lethargy,
- low blood sugar,
- migraines,
- mood swings,
- muscle and joint pains,
- panic attacks,
- poor concentration,
- poor digestion,
- sciatica,
- spontaneous abortion,
- spontaneous bruising,
- stiffness,
- thinning hair,
- water retention.

Similar claims, of course, were made when estrogen was
first introduced. It was only twenty years later that ques-

tions arose about the possible side effects. The whole history of health and medicine demonstrates the wisdom of scepticism about any ''wonder'' substance that hits the headlines. I am suspicious about anything that is claimed to cure such a wide range of symptoms. And what is so ''natural'' about the idea of women taking progesterone? As explained in Chapter 1, production of both estrogen and progesterone declines at the menopause. And although we go on making some estrogen all our lives, the production of progesterone will stop completely. So are we seriously suggesting that nature has got this all wrong? At a time in our lives when both hormones are dropping and progesterone can be absent, why should we be adding it back in? Progesterone is needed to maintain a pregnancy, so we can understand why the body doesn't need it at the menopause. Why replace it?

What, actually, could be more unnatural than doctoring ourselves with progesterone, when Mother Nature has arranged for its removal from the body in the normal course of events? The thinking behind the growing popularity of progesterone therapy is as follows. As inhabitants of an industrialized world, we are being constantly bombarded by xenoestrogens—substances that have an estrogenic effect on the body. These xenoestrogens are nearly all petrochemically based and can come from packaging, plastics, foods, and pesticides. They have been found in formula baby milk, assumed to have originated from the packaging used to contain the milk. They are believed to have a devastating effect on fertility, reproduction, and health for both humans and wildlife. A number of disturbing developments are increasingly blamed on these chemicals. In the West it is reckoned that men's sperm count may have dropped by 50 percent in the last ten years. Other studies have linked these chemicals to the increase in breast and testicular cancers and to endometriosis, a painful uterine disorder. This major environmental factor lies behind the theory of *estrogen dominance*.

The suggestion is that many of us are suffering from estrogen dominance because of the increased number of xenoestrogens we encounter daily. So, the argument goes, the answer is to balance all this unwanted estrogen with progesterone—natural progesterone. I believe that our life-styles and our environment have a profound effect on our hormones. That is why we must take a lot of care over our nutrition, which has such an impact on the body's biochemical processes. I don't, however, believe that the answer is to introduce ever more hormones into our bodies. And the question we should ask is, just how "natural" is progesterone anyway?

Progesterone has a long history. It was originally obtained from sows' ovaries, and in the late 1930s it could be synthesized from placentas in large amounts. So placentas were quick-frozen after delivery for later extraction of progesterone. After a number of years a way was found of converting diosgenin from the wild yam (*Dioscorea villosa*) into progesterone. This diosgenin became the starting point in the chemical manufacturing process of progesterone, which was converted to the synthetic progesterone first used in birth control pills and later in Hormone Replacement Therapy. Because progesterone is a fat-soluble compound, it was usually ineffective when taken by mouth because it was metabolized by the liver and never got into the blood-stream in sufficient amounts. This led to progesterone being given intramuscularly by injection and also as a suppository inserted into the vagina or rectum. It has been used for many years in this way as a treatment for premenstrual syndrome. It is now available in the form of cream to rub on the surface of the skin and is sold in the United States over the counter as a cosmetic. In Britain it is sold by prescription only, which upsets many of its advocates. They claim that because the progesterone is "natural" it is safe to use and should be available over the counter.

This "natural" progesterone is often thought of as an extract from wild yam. In fact, progesterone itself is not found in wild yams. It is synthesized from the plant by a number of chemical steps, which means that it is not "natural" at all. The assumption was that if we ate wild yam, our bodies could convert it into the biologically active human hormone progesterone. This is simply not true. Although progesterone can be synthesized from diosgenin, it can be done only by a chemist in a laboratory. Our bodies are just not capable of synthesizing progesterone from a substance such as wild yam. We do not have the necessary enzymatic pathways to produce this conversion. And the fact is that these progesterone creams *do not contain any wild yam at all*, a fact confirmed by Dr. John Lee, the California physician who has written most widely about it. As the demand for progesterone grew, the wild yam became overharvested, and other sources had to be found. Now the main manufacturers use soybeans instead. The creams are fortified with the addition of USP-grade progesterone, a white powder that used to be derived from wild yam and is now more often derived from soybeans. Progesterone is called "natural progesterone" to identify it as being chemically identical to the progesterone produced by humans and to differentiate it from the synthetic progestogen used in HRT.

Why, anyway, should a progesterone supplement or replacement be necessary? Cholesterol is the starting block (the precursor) of progesterone and all the other sex hormones in our bodies. As most of us know, the worry has usually been that we have too much cholesterol in our diet. So the difficulty is not that we have some undesirable shortage of this progesterone starting block but that our hormonal pathways necessary for this conversion start to shut down.

You need to be aware that progesterone creams contain a powerful pharmaceutical hormone which is made in a laboratory. Because the FDA (Food and Drug Administration) won't allow the manufacturers of the creams to make medical claims, they are sold as cosmetics, not as hormone replacements. It is because these creams contain a pharmaceutical agent that the British Medicines Control Agency will let them be sold only under prescription, and rightly so. My main concern is that women are being duped into thinking they are buying a natural herbal remedy containing wild yam. They are not: they are buying hormone replacement—just a different hormone (progesterone instead of the usual HRT combination of a form of estrogen plus progestogen). And they may not be buying anything truly to do with wild yam, which has a very respectable reputation as a herbal treatment for menstrual and menopausal problems. Although for centuries herbalists have indeed used wild yam in a tincture form, the effect of the herb in its pure state is very different from that of the synthesized progesterone. This wild yam is taken orally and has traditionally been used as an anti-spasmodic and anti-inflammatory herb. As is the case with so many effective herbs, it is not known precisely how it acts on the body. Since the essence of herbal medicine is that all the ingredients help toward the overall therapeutic effect, diosgenin alone cannot be responsible for the wild yam's beneficial qualities. Herbs work because they contain a host of substances—active substances, balancing substances, and substances that cope with any side effects of the active substances. They are holistic and truly "natural." But the "natural" progesterone that is being hyped is no more "natural" than a number of the plant-based estrogen preparations that form the basis of some HRT products.

These estrogens are "natural" in the same sense that plant-based progesterone is classed as "natural." The estrogens, too, are synthesized in the laboratory from soybeans and yams. They still have side effects, however. We need to be clear that these hormones, estrogen and progesterone, which are synthesized in a laboratory from plants, are not natural to us. They may be chemically identical to what our bodies produce, but they are powerful drugs—hence the need to put them on prescription. Plant-based progesterone is termed "natural" because it has the same molecular structure as the progesterone molecule found in humans. This idea of different substances being chemically identical can be very misleading. For example, coal, diamond, and graphite (the "lead" in your pencil) are all chemically identical, and yet they have very different properties and functions. They have the same molecular structure, but you wouldn't expect to produce much heat by putting diamonds on the fire.

You may have heard that progesterone can help menopausal symptoms and protect you from osteoporosis. The same question that is asked about HRT would have to be asked in progesterone's case also: when do you stop taking it? According to Dr. John Lee, the answer is, "Do it until you are ninety-six and then we will reconsider."[1] You will not be the same at seventy as you are at fifty-six, so how do you know how much to use? Are you estrogen dominant (that is, over-supplied with estrogen), or are your hormones doing what they are supposed to at that age anyway? Yes, you can have your hormones tested and know what the profile is, but if you then continued to use progesterone cream for years, you would need to keep having tests to know whether you were overdosing or not. It's all a bit hit and miss.

The cream is rubbed into the skin so it can be absorbed directly into the bloodstream.[2] A team of researchers in Belgium found that the cream tended to accumulate in the skin instead of being fully absorbed into the bloodstream. Dr. Lee advises applying the cream on a rotational basis to different parts of the body. You can imagine that if you use the cream for forty years, from the menopause to age ninety-six as he suggests, you will have used all the possible sites available, and it is unknown what the side effects of the hormone accumulation in the fat cells will be. Dr. Lee also believes that during the initial stages of being used, the cream temporarily sensitizes the body to estrogen. It is estrogen sensitivity that has been linked to breast and endometrial cancers, fibroids, and endometriosis. So by using progesterone cream are you increasing the risks of disease? And progesterone has some well-known side effects. In the *British National Formulary* (*BNF*), which many British doctors keep in their offices, progesterone is listed separately from progestogens. And according to the *BNF* the side effects of progesterone include acne, urticaria, fluid retention, weight changes, gastrointestinal disturbances, changes in libido, breast discomfort, and menstrual irregularities. Claims have been put forward that progesterone can protect against breast cancer, although there are arguments that higher levels of progesterone may be a risk factor for breast cancer.[3] In animal studies, cancer of the ovary, uterus, and breast were all linked to increased progesterone.[4]

Even Dr. Lee admits that women taking "natural" progesterone may experience exaggerated pre-menstrual or menopausal symptoms at the beginning. There are possibilities of breakthrough bleeding (bleeding that occurs at times in the cycle other than during a period) and other cycle irregularities also. Linda, who is forty-seven, came to see me after using a progesterone cream over a period of two months. She had been advised to use it even though she had had no menopausal symptoms and was still getting regular periods. She then started to get breakthrough bleeding halfway through the month. She was obviously concerned about this but was told that it was "normal" and that her body would adjust. The bleeding continued, so she decided to stop using the cream. At this point, she was overwhelmed by hot flashes and tiredness which she had not had before. Linda was getting hot all over, and waking up during the night; then she would feel really cold. She had lost her sex drive and felt "very fed up." By this time she had not had a period for six weeks, which was very unusual for her. Obviously she was worried. I recommended a good nutritional program tailored to her needs and herbs to redress the imbalance. By the time she returned in a month, the hot flashes had gone, her energy was back, and her periods had returned. I felt that the progesterone had had a pronounced effect on her hormone levels and it was only through a more gentle, natural approach that her body was able to balance itself.

It is true that Dr. Lee's research appears to demonstrate that progesterone cream has improved bone density among his patients who could not take estrogen therapy. But his admirable desire to help those women who could not take HRT leaves a fundamental question mark over the results of his surveys, since it means there is no "control" group not taking progesterone whose results could be compared. The British Natural Osteoporosis Society (NOS) marks its concern by stating that there has been "little validated scientific research into the effects of progesterone alone on bone density or fracture risk." NOS medical advisers do not recommend the use of "natural progesterone" creams to prevent osteoporosis (or to counteract the effect of estrogen in HRT products). Their recommendations for healthy bones include a well-balanced diet, regular exercise, no smoking, and a minimal intake of alcohol. Dr. Lee also made recommendations on exercise, diet, and nutrient supplements as part of the treatment. It could well be that these factors, rather than the progesterone itself, were responsible for the improvement in his patients.

This is very important. My main fear is that the media hype about progesterone and the desire for easy solutions to myriad complaints are obscuring the real issues. Are we merely falling into the same trap that we did in the fifties and sixties when estrogen was hailed as the wonder cure for menopausal women? First we try one hormone and then another. First it was estrogen. Now it's progesterone. Both, I believe, are short-sighted, short-term solutions which may have long-term negative effects. Surely the aim is to get our bodies back in balance naturally—and to allow our bodies to do this themselves. By adding in any kind of direct hormone we are never addressing the fundamental cause of problems. If you stop the cream, you are back to square one: your body will not have become any healthier in the process.

There is the possibility, too, that supplying something from an outside source merely encourages the body to produce less of its own. This is known to happen when people are given the thyroid hormone thyroxin. Our bodies are extremely clever. Why produce something yourself when it is being supplied from the outside and somebody else can do the work! And can it be sensible for women to take progesterone supplements after the menopause when the body's own production of the hormone stops quite naturally? Its fans talk of progesterone as the "missing" hormone. But after a certain stage of our lives it's not supposed to be there anyway.

"Natural" progesterone is being touted as a "natural" alternative to HRT. But there is nothing natural or alternative about it. The theory behind it is the same as the theory behind HRT—that menopausal women are suffering from a hormone deficiency disorder, a modern complaint that has arisen because we are now living way beyond our reproductive years. That is how the medical establishment, when pressed, explains and justifies the case for hormone supplementation.

The whole approach of this book is to get you healthy naturally so that your body has the capability to balance your hormones naturally. You change your nutrition, you add in food supplements (substances you would normally eat but which perhaps you need in more concentrated forms for a while), your digestion and absorption are improved. Herbal medicine, acupuncture, and homeopathy can be used where appropriate. The result is a state of good health and balance. Isn't this really the best way forward?

It was almost twenty years before it was realized that estrogen replacement therapy had increased the risk of endometrial cancer dramatically. Are we going to have to wait another twenty years for the progesterone time-bomb to explode, after we have all been used as human guinea pigs?

CHAPTER 5

Best nutrition for the menopause

The best-kept secret of good health during the menopause is to eat as naturally as possible. Good nutrition means not only eating the "right" foods but also avoiding the "bad" ones. So where do you begin? Let's start by exploding a myth. There are no such things as "health" or "healthy" foods. This is just marketing hype. There are foods that are *not* good for you and there are foods that are *natural*. Natural foods are those that your body can digest easily and use to maximum benefit. Those are the foods that your body needs in order to be able to respond naturally to the different stages of your life.

In computer jargon there is a saying, GIGO, which stands for "Garbage In, Garbage Out." In other words, you get *out* only as good as you put *in*. If you put poor-quality gas in a high-performance car like a Rolls-Royce or a Cadillac it may run for a while, but eventually it will become less productive and less efficient. It will probably start to run down until the engine deteriorates so much it can no longer work. It is exactly the same with the human body. You need top-grade "fuel" to function properly. Survival is your body's top priority, and it will use whatever nourishment you give it to try to keep healthy. However, you can make this job either much harder, by providing poor-quality food and drink, which will eventually lead to bad health, or much easier, by providing a quality diet, which will keep you feeling healthy, fit, and well.

Good nutrition is essential during the menopause so that your body can adjust itself automatically and keep your hormones in balance, thus avoiding or preventing disease. (Dis-ease means not being at ease or being out of balance).

If you can keep your body in balance and allow your own hormones to work to the optimum during these menopausal years, and naturally maintain estrogen from the adrenals and fat deposits, you have a much better chance of reducing the symptoms of the menopause to the minimum or even avoiding them altogether.

The eating plan outlined in this chapter is an enjoyable, pleasurable, and healthy way of eating. It is not a diet that you follow for a short while and then abandon for your former unhealthful eating patterns. It is easy to follow on a daily basis, full of variety, and very tasty. I know this because I eat this way myself.

There may be occasions when it is not possible to follow the guidelines—perhaps when you are being entertained by others; but so long as your foundation of eating is good, these exceptions will not make much difference. Above all, food is to be enjoyed. Eating is a time for sharing and socializing. Remember: this is not a strict diet but a plan for making improvements in your eating patterns to enhance your health and well-being.

Some changes are fairly easy to make—such as choosing free-range eggs or drinking diluted fruit juice instead of soda pop. Others may be harder—such as giving up coffee, tea, and sugary snacks. Don't be put off because you think altering your eating habits sounds too difficult. Try taking it one step at a time. You'll be pleasantly surprised at how well you can adapt to changes if you make them gradually. Once you start to feel the benefits, you'll know that it was all worthwhile. Even if you are not able to make all the changes suggested, do what you can. As one of my clients, Sally, found, it is amazing how even a small improvement can go a long way toward easing the symptoms.

Sally came to see me when she was forty-one because she was determined to do all she could to prevent the symptoms of the menopause. She wanted to get herself as well as possible, to learn what to eat and drink and what to avoid. She also wanted to know what supplements, if any, would be good to take. She was looking for good general advice on how she could prepare for the menopause. Sally had a few minor symptoms such as headaches behind the eyes and low back pain. Her doctor had been suggesting she take HRT, because although she was still having regular periods they were very heavy. She had been feeling some heat at night but none during the day.

At first I recommended that she try to cut back on tea, coffee, and sugary foods. She soon noticed the benefits. Her energy levels increased, and she was sleeping better because she was not feeling hot at night. Sally was so cheered by the results that she asked what else she could do. I advised her that she should start to check the labels on foods in order to eliminate added sugar, preservatives, additives, etc., and to buy brands free of these "additions" where possible. She also increased her intake of fresh fruit and vegetables and cut down on the amount of processed and convenience foods she was eating.

When we reviewed all the changes that she had made, Sally was surprised at how easy it had been to adapt to her new eating pattern. She says that if she had been faced with such an upheaval in one go, she might have found it overwhelming. It was because she took it gradually, progressing from one step to the next in her own time as she felt the benefits, that she was encouraged to keep it up.

We all have very different eating patterns, depending on personal preferences and our lifestyles. However, there are certain steps that every woman can take to try to improve her health during the menopause:

❑ Stabilize blood sugar levels by reducing your input of refined foods and those foods and drinks that have a stimulant effect; eat regular amounts of complex carbohydrates and fresh fruit.

❑ Avoid tea, coffee, and alcohol—addictive drinks— which contribute to the blood sugar level problem and also deprive the body of vital nutrients and trace elements.

❑ Reduce your intake of dairy products and red meat, which can adversely affect your health during the menopause.

❑ Ensure that your diet contains sufficient essential fatty acids and a minimum of non-essential fats.

❑ Check that you are eating enough fiber from natural sources.
❑ Reduce your intake of sodium.

This chapter aims to help you make any necessary changes by explaining how different foods and drinks affect your body. Once you understand these effects, you can take control of your health. You will know what and when to eat to ensure optimum well-being during the menopausal years.

Some of the physiological functions explained can be quite technical, so I have made a simple summary of recommendations at the end of each heading. The chapter concludes with practical advice on reading food labels and on cooking and preparing foods and a suggested shopping list of foods and drinks you should include and those you should avoid during the menopause.

Stabilize your blood sugar levels

Maintaining a steady blood sugar level can make a big difference in how you feel emotionally and physically before, during, and after the menopause. A healthy blood sugar balance will enable the female hormones you have circulating to be fully utilized, which will help you to avoid many of the unpleasant symptoms you might otherwise experience.

Nutrition is the key to stabilizing your level of blood sugar (glucose). Glucose is the only form in which food can be absorbed by the body and turned into energy. After a meal, glucose from the breakdown of food (digestion) is absorbed through the wall of the intestine into the bloodstream. At this point, there is a high level of glucose in the blood, so the body produces insulin from the pancreas in an attempt to lower the level. Any extra glucose, which is not used for energy, is changed into glycogen and stored in the liver and muscles. The glucose level in the blood then reduces to normal.

Your body works in a similar way to the thermostat on your heating system to balance the blood sugar level.

❏ When in balance your body maintains its own optimum blood glucose levels.

❏ *When the glucose level rises too high*, insulin is produced to lower it. If the blood sugar level remains too high, this causes the symptoms of hyperglycemia—high blood sugar level. The extreme form of hyperglycemia is diabetes. With this condition, insulin is supplied from outside the body by injection to bring the level down.

❏ *When the glucose level falls too low*, the hormone adrenaline is released from the adrenal glands and glucagon is produced from the pancreas. Glucagon works in the opposite way to insulin and increases blood glucose by encouraging the liver to turn some of its glycogen stores into glucose.

  If the blood glucose level stays low for a period of time, this can cause symptoms of hypoglycemia—low blood sugar level. These symptoms, which include irritability, aggressive outbursts, palpitations, forgetfulness, lack of sex drive, and excess sweating, have a marked similarity to those associated with hormone imbalance experienced during premenstrual syndrome and the menopause.

During a normal day, the amount by which your blood sugar level rises and falls depends on two main factors:

❏ what you have had to eat or drink
❏ when you last ate or drank.

WHAT YOU EAT OR DRINK

All the food you eat is broken down into glucose. When you eat any food in refined form (sugar, chocolate, white flour, candy, cookies, cake), digestion is very fast, and glucose enters the body rapidly. Any food or drink that causes a stimulant effect, such as tea, coffee, alcohol, chocolate, sugar, or candy, affects your blood sugar level and causes a sharp and fast rise in the blood glucose, followed by a rapid drop. Smoking has the same effect.

At this low point, you feel tired and drained and need

something like a candy bar or cup of coffee (or both!) to give you a boost. This boost causes the blood sugar level to go up rapidly, and the cycle is repeated. All of this causes an up-and-down, roller-coaster ride of blood sugar swings.

Over time, this constant over-stimulation exhausts the pancreas. Now, instead of too much insulin, it produces too little. Too much glucose stays in the blood, causing the symptoms of high blood sugar levels.

WHEN YOU EAT OR DRINK

If there is a long gap since your last food (over three hours in women), your blood glucose will drop to quite a low level. You can then feel the need for a quick boost (cup of coffee, cookie). At the same time, the adrenal glands will make the liver produce more glucose. The combination of these two causes high levels of glucose in the blood, which again calls on the pancreas to overproduce insulin in order to reduce the glucose levels. The roller-coaster ride starts all over again, and the adrenal glands become more exhausted.

Effects of adrenaline

If blood sugar levels are repeatedly low and adrenaline is pumped into the body on a regular basis, this can take a toll on your health, especially during the menopause.

Adrenaline is the hormone most of us associate with stress. It is the hormone that is released for "fight or flight" and its effect is very powerful. The heart speeds up and the arteries tighten to raise blood pressure. The liver immediately releases emergency stores of glucose—instant energy—into the bloodstream. Digestion stops because it is not necessary for survival and the clotting ability of the blood is increased in case of injury. This all means that we are prepared to run faster, fight back, react more quickly than normal.

Unfortunately when our blood sugar level drops during the day or night, adrenaline is released automatically, and the body experiences all the above sensations except that there is no outside stress to respond to. When this happens repeatedly, we can see the effect on our health and the part it plays in heart disease (increased clotting of the blood, higher blood pressure) and extreme fluctuations of sugar levels caused by the release of sugar to give us energy.

Repeated stimulation of the adrenal glands can interfere with their proper functioning. During the menopause, it is crucial that your adrenal glands be working at their optimum and not become exhausted because of the extra work they are having to do. At this time of a woman's life, the adrenal glands are required to produce estrogen, since the ovaries are producing less and less. The adrenal glands also produce a natural hormone, DHEA (dehydroepiandrosterone), which has been linked to anti-aging.

Clearly, maintaining blood sugar levels is an important factor in good health at the time of the menopause. This can be achieved by careful consideration not only of what you eat and drink, but also of *when* you eat and drink.

How can these highs and lows be prevented?

1. Regular intake of complex carbohydrates

Dr. Katharina Dalton, a pioneer in the recognition and treatment of premenstrual syndrome (PMS), has found that one way the symptoms of PMS and the menopause can be relieved is by eating regularly. This stops the blood sugar level from dropping and adrenaline from being released. You are ideally looking for foods that give you a slow rise in blood sugar and keep the level up for about three hours. You can then eat again before it drops.

Complex carbohydrates are the best foods for this. They give a slow release of energy because it takes time for the digestive tract to break them down into the simplest substances that the body can use. Carbohydrates are a large group of foods which include sugars and starches. They are an important source of energy and are all eventually broken down in the body into the simple sugar, glucose. It is the speed with which this happens that is the important factor. There are two types of carbohydrates: complex and simple.

To help maintain a steady blood sugar level, aim to eat

Complex carbohydrates	Simple carbohydrates
Grains (wheat, rye, oats, rice, barley, corn)	Fruit
	Honey
	White and brown sugar
Beans (lentils, kidney beans, chickpeas, aduki beans, haricot beans, etc.)	Glucose in "high energy" drinks
Vegetables	
Fiber in grains, beans, and vegetables	

complex carbohydrates regularly during the day. You do not necessarily need to eat more. Sometimes just a wholewheat cracker can be enough between meals. If you find that the symptoms associated with low blood sugar levels are greatest first thing in the morning or if you wake during the night, heart pounding, and cannot get back to sleep, it is very likely that your blood sugar level has dropped overnight and adrenaline has kicked into play. Eating a small, starchy snack one hour before going to bed (e.g. a cracker) and, if possible, one hour after getting up will help to alleviate these symptoms.

Whenever possible, choose unrefined complex carbohydrates such as wholewheat bread, brown rice, and wholewheat flour. When a carbohydrate is refined, the food is stripped of essential vitamins, minerals, trace elements, and its valuable fiber content. It was originally thought that fiber's role was only to speed up the passage of digested food to prevent constipation. It is now known that some forms of fiber can actually slow down the absorption of sugars and help to maintain our blood sugar balance. Without fiber, food acts more quickly on the blood sugar level and is harder to eliminate from the body.

Eating the right foods regularly—i.e., complex carbohydrates every three hours—can stop cravings and binges on foods that appear to offer a "kick start" but only bring associated health problems. Shelagh, thirty-nine, came to see me with terrible migraines which occurred around the time of her period—either the day before, on the day the period started, or the day after. She got flashing lights, and tended to feel very sick with it. She craved sweet cookies and kept a bag of them with her all the time so she could nibble when she felt the need. After the pain had gone she craved junk food. Shelagh said she had a "dreadful craving" for chocolate.

I suggested that for the first two months she start to eat starchy foods every three hours, to keep her blood sugar levels steady. By keeping her blood sugar level in balance, she would then stop any drastic drops in sugar levels and hence reduce the sugar cravings. After the first two months she came back saying she felt much better, had more energy, and did not have her usual premenstrual agitation. She had not had any weekend headaches, which had been a regular pattern before.

Shelagh said that her food cravings had almost gone. She occasionally felt she wanted something, but there was now no compulsion. These changes were not due to willpower; her body just did not need those large amounts of sugar-rich food, so she had no cravings to eat it. She told me, "I've been eating every three hours and do feel better for it—no shakes and tension through lack of food! I had some of the migraine symptoms during my period but was not incapacitated as I usually am."

I then suggested some food supplements to balance her deficiencies as suggested by the health questionnaire she had completed. She wrote the next month, "I actually got through this month with no migraine! Only the warning signs, so I'm very cheered." A couple of months later she dropped me a line to say, "I haven't had a full migraine for two months although I'm still getting the aura symptoms. Thank you for all your help!"

If you experience binges and cravings, these may indicate a blood sugar imbalance as described above. They may also be symptoms of a food allergy, so this is worth checking. Ironically, if we are allergic to or intolerant of a particular food, we tend to crave it and eat it more. Ask yourself the question "Which foods or drinks would I find hard to give up?" That will give you a clue to what to look out for.

2. Avoidance of refined foods, especially sugar

It is better to avoid the simple carbohydrates, where possible, except fruit. Although fruit contains fructose (fruit sugar), which is a simple sugar, the fiber content of the fruit is a complex carbohydrate which slows the digestion rate. So fructose is acceptable when taken in the whole fruit, like an apple, but not when used in the refined form of powdered white fructose. Pure fruit juice can also cause a rapid change in blood sugar level because it is not buffered by the fiber that is normally present. It is better to dilute fruit juice to make it less concentrated.

A can of cola may contain up to eight teaspoons of sugar, as may a tub of fruit yogurt. Most of the convenience foods and drinks we buy are laden with sugar. Sugar is also in non-sweet foods such as ketchup, baked beans, and mayonnaise. Indeed, sugar is added to practically everything, as it is an inexpensive bulking agent. Even some toothpastes contain sugar. Because toothpaste is not a food, this does not have to be put on the ingredients list.

When sugar is in its natural form—the whole sugar cane—it is fine to eat. It has all the right amounts of fiber and is a whole food. The problem starts when it is refined. The processing and refinement removes the fiber as well as the vitamins, minerals, and trace elements. The same is true for white flour. In order to digest these refined foods your body has to use its own vitamins and minerals, so depleting your own stores.

You may be tempted to substitute artificial sweeteners for sugar; don't. You are simply substituting a chemical which is alien to the body and has to be dealt with, giving it extra work to do. Nobody really knows what havoc these chemicals can cause when introduced to your body's own delicately balanced biochemistry. If a food or drink is described as "low sugar" or "diet," it will usually contain a chemical sweetener. Artificial sweeteners are also found in some potato chips, juice pops, sauces, pot noodles and some medicines (check the label carefully). There is more information about artificial sweeteners in the section on reading labels (see page 68).

3. Reducing foods and drinks that are stimulants

Stimulants in your diet (alcohol, sugar, nicotine from smoking, and caffeine in tea, coffee, and chocolate) cause a fast rise in your blood sugar levels, followed by a fast drop, which contributes to the roller-coaster ride of blood sugar swings. They can actually increase hot flashes by causing the blood vessels to dilate. Just hot drinks themselves can worsen hot flashes. When we drink something hot on a summer's day, it has a cooling effect by dilating the blood vessels and allowing us to sweat more through the skin. Indeed, you may have noticed the connection between a cup of tea or coffee and the start of a hot flash. The same is true for spicy foods such as curries, so keep these to a minimum during the menopause.

Avoid addictive drinks

Alcohol, tea, and coffee are called "social poisons"—socially acceptable drugs which have an antidepressant or stimulant effect. Because they are socially acceptable we tend to forget their addictive properties. However, during the menopause it is especially important to look at the effects on your health and then ask yourself, is it worth it?

When we are younger, we are adaptable, flexible, and able to eliminate toxins more easily. Eventually, as we grow older and the effects accumulate, our bodies rebel, seeming to say: "If you keep putting this rubbish in me, I will just get slower, sicker, and look and feel older than my years." As teenagers we could get away with it; as we grow older our bodies have less tolerance.

COFFEE

Coffee contains three stimulants—caffeine, theobromine, and theophylline. A cup of instant coffee contains around

---

Recommendations for stabilizing your blood sugar levels

Include:
- Unrefined complex carbohydrates such as whole-wheat bread, whole-wheat meal pasta, potatoes, brown rice, millet, oats, rye.
- Eat fruits and drink diluted pure fruit juice.
- Always eat breakfast—oats are good.
- Eat small, frequent meals.

Avoid:
- Refined carbohydrates, such as white flour in cakes, cookies, pastries.
- Tea, coffee (also decaffeinated, as it contains two other stimulants), alcohol.
- Sugar and foods containing sugar (chocolate, candies, cookies).
- Soft drinks.
- Convenience foods, as they are likely to contain refined carbohydrates.
- Smoking.

66mg. of caffeine. Filtered coffee contains even more.

The diuretic effect of caffeine may flush vital nutrients and trace elements out of the body. Added to this problem, the active ingredients in caffeine, called methylxanthines, have been linked to a benign breast disease known as fibrocystic disease. Many women experience breast discomfort in the week before a period which can become worse as they reach their forties and can develop into mastalgia. The pain can be very intense and at over forty years of age can occur at any time of the month. By cutting out coffee, women have found relief from mastalgia. Because these methylxanthines are in caffeine, chocolate, cola drinks, cocoa and tea are also culprits. Although decaffeinated coffee does not contain caffeine, it still contains theobromine and theophylline, which can disturb normal sleep patterns. Also, most decaffeinated coffee has often been decaffeinated by a chemical process.

TEA

Tea contains both caffeine (around 50mg. per cup) and tannin. All the above effects of caffeine still apply. Tannin binds important minerals and prevents their absorption in the digestive tract. At this stage in your life, when you need to maximize your intake of such important minerals as calcium, zinc, iron, magnesium, etc., it is essential that you do not prevent them from being absorbed. Otherwise it could get to a stage where you are eating a nutritious diet, perhaps even taking vitamin and mineral supplements, and yet at the same time these vital nutrients are wasted because they are being excreted, rather than absorbed.

ALCOHOL

Although the consumption of alcohol in the United States has actually declined slightly in recent years, alcohol is still a contributor to many health problems. Alcohol is full of calories. It is made by the action of yeast on sugar, so provides these calories in the form of a carbohydrate. One 6 oz. (180 ml.) glass of wine provides us with 150 calories and 12 oz. (355 ml.) of beer around 145 calories.

As we have already seen, alcohol can contribute to a low blood sugar problem. It can also cause liver damage. Furthermore, it acts as an anti-nutrient: that is, it blocks the good effects of our food by depleting the body of vitamins and minerals, especially zinc. Alcohol interferes with your metabolism of essential fatty acids, which are needed to produce prostaglandins, chemicals that help to control moods, immunity, and vascular reactions such as hot flashes.

Thankfully, more and more people are now becoming aware of the health problems associated with these addictive drinks and are turning to alternatives. However, as with all drugs, there can be withdrawal symptoms when you stop. These include: headaches, nausea, tiredness, and depression. The withdrawal symptoms can be quite dramatic. Some hospitals have now discovered that certain postoperative symptoms are not caused by the effects of anesthetic, as previously thought, but by caffeine withdrawal. Before a general anesthetic, patients are asked not to eat or drink for a number of hours; and by the time they come around from the operation the withdrawal symptoms have already started.

To minimize these effects, cut down slowly, substituting some of your usual drinks for alternatives. I gave up coffee a few years ago and did not do it gradually. I had a migraine-like headache and the "shakes," which lasted for about three days. Several patients of mine have experienced pains in their legs after giving up coffee, but they felt they could "see light at the end of the tunnel" and persevered and have felt so much better since. As in the case of Sue, forty-five, who came to see me complaining of headaches and dizziness.

Sue was experiencing anxiety and panic attacks and said she felt muzzy and tired all the time. The panic attacks would come on suddenly, and she would feel hot and start sweating. This would also be accompanied by palpitations. She sometimes woke in the night with them. Her mother had been fifty when she started the menopause, so Sue was obviously keen to get herself really well before this age.

Some years before, Sue had begun to have very heavy periods, sometimes only a week apart. A fibroid the size of a coconut had been found, so a hysterectomy was recommended. Her left tube and ovary were also removed. She had been put on HRT (Premarin), but the headaches were so excruciating she had to stop. She was then switched to estrogen patches and was on them when she came to see me. Sue was also keen to come off the medication she was taking for the panic attacks.

Her answers to my health questionnaire (see page 218) showed that Sue was drinking eight cups of coffee a day and four cups of tea. I suggested that we aim to cut these out completely, bringing her intake down gradually each day and substituting some herbal teas or grain coffees. Sue felt that her personality was such that if she knew something was not good for her she would rather get rid of it now, once and for all.

So she stopped both tea and coffee on a Monday. By Tuesday she had started to suffer terrible headaches, and on Wednesday night began to have cramps. Sue persevered, and within a week the headaches and cramps had gone. She said she was amazed at the extent of the withdrawal symptoms: she would never have believed it if she hadn't gone through them. When she came back to see me, she had checked with her doctor that it was all right to stop her medication abruptly, and so she came off the HRT and the medicine for her panic attacks.

Another patient who benefited enormously from giving up coffee and tea is Joy, who was fifty-six when she first came to see me. She was still menstruating, but over the last few months the pattern of her cycle had become very worrying. Her periods had become increasingly heavy, and in one period Joy started to hemorrhage. She was put on HRT and the hemorrhaging stopped, but she said she felt so tired and depressed on the HRT.

Eventually Joy saw a gynecologist, who suggested she have a hysterectomy, because he had discovered a fibroid. Fibroids can cause excessive bleeding and may also delay the onset of the menopause. But once the menopause arrives, fibroids start to shrink because of the lack of female hormones and are not usually a problem any more. So Joy was in a catch-22 situation. Her fibroids were delaying the menopause, yet if she could get through the menopause it was unlikely she would need the hysterectomy, as the fibroids would go. She told the gynecologist that she would like to try another approach, so he delayed the hysterectomy for six months, and in the meantime she came to see me.

I explained to Joy that coffee was a definite culprit in terms of excess bleeding and fibroids. She changed to herbal teas and grain coffee and found that the bleeding stopped. I also recommended some herbs to help balance her female hormones. By the time Joy had been to see me a couple of times, her heavy bleeding had become just regular periods, and she found she bled excessively or between

Recommendations for avoiding addictive drinks

Reduce:
• Coffee, tea, and alcohol.

Substitute and include:
• Instant grain "coffees"—Bambu, Kaffree Roma, Cafix.
• Herb teas, fruit teas—Luaka, Japanese twig (bancha) tea.
• Pure fruit juice diluted with sparkling mineral water; sparkling apple juice—After the Fall, Martinelli.

periods only if she drank coffee or was under a lot of stress.

She went back to the gynecologist three months after her first visit to me. He gave her an internal check and said that everything was fine; her womb was not enlarged and the fibroids were slightly smaller. Since the bleeding was now under control, she could postpone the hysterectomy indefinitely. Within a year she let me know that her periods had stopped completely, and she was very grateful to have kept her body intact.

Reduce your intake of dairy products and red meat

In the Western world we eat far more protein than we really need. Excess protein has been linked to kidney stones, gout, and high blood pressure. A certain amount of protein is essential. Proteins are the building blocks in our food. They are necessary for the structural formation of our bones, skin, hair, and muscle. However, it is important to monitor our intake of protein to ensure not only that we are getting the correct amount but also that it is coming from the most healthful sources.

Red meat, which includes beef, pork, and game, should be omitted completely. Red meat worsens estrogen deficiency. Because it is high in phosphates, it increases the loss of calcium from the bones, thereby increasing the risk of osteoporosis.

Poultry and eggs should be bought with care. Choose free-range, which have been produced without the use of growth promoters, antibiotics, or hormones. It is hard enough to balance our own hormones without introducing extra ones given to animals. Make sure that all chicken is thoroughly cooked to kill off any bacteria.

Dairy products should be used sparingly, as they contain casein, the protein in cheese, milk, and cream, which is not assimilated by many people. Casein is three hundred times higher in cows' milk than human milk, as it is important for the fast development of large bones in calves.

Cows' milk is not designed for human consumption. The cow has a four-stomach digestive system, which can deal with the casein easily. But it cannot easily be absorbed by humans, so milk remains undigested in the gut and begins to putrefy and rot. This putrefaction in humans produces toxins and mucus. It clings as undigested matter to the lining of the intestines and prevents the absorption of vital nutrients into the body.

This digestive struggle takes a lot of energy to sort out. That means that the energy you would have to enjoy life and do the things you want is now being spent sorting out your digestion. The result is that you feel tired. How many times have you felt sleepy after a meal? Your body is using much more energy than it should to digest the food. When you feel like that it may be worth looking at what you have eaten. Dairy produce (i.e. milk, butter, and cheese) can also cause a runny nose, catarrh, a feeling that you need to clear your throat, and a host of other unpleasant symptoms.

Clare had been suffering from shaking, anxiety, palpitations, sweating, and insomnia. She found herself crying for no particular reason and felt she was becoming agoraphobic, not wanting to go out and socialize. She also had high blood pressure and had been put on Bendrofluazide, although this had not reduced her blood pressure at all. Her blood pressure was as high as 150/100. (A normal blood

---

Recommendations for reducing your consumption of red meat and dairy products

Include:
- Fish, poultry, eggs.
- Organic goats' or cows' milk in moderation. (If you suspect an allergy, consult a good nutritional therapist.)
- Live, natural yogurt with lactobacillus acidophilus.
- Nuts, seeds, grains, beans, tofu.

Avoid:
- Beef, pork, and game.

---

pressure is around 120/80 with individual variations.)

Clare told me that her grandfather had died of a heart attack, so she was very keen to find the cause of the high blood pressure and do something about it. Because her blood pressure had not been reduced by the medication, I felt that something external must be to blame. I suggested that she cut out dairy foods (high saturated-fat content) and have her blood pressure monitored to see if there were any changes.

A month later she came back to report that the change had been remarkable. Her blood pressure was now down to 120/80. She had tried introducing dairy foods back into her diet and had immediately gotten a tight feeling in her chest and the return of her old symptoms, including giddiness. I devised a program of supplements for her to make sure she was getting all the necessary nutrients, and she said she felt so much better and hadn't fully appreciated how stressed she had been feeling in the past.

An added problem with dairy produce is what the farmers are giving their cows. They are now fed antibiotics to speed their growth, other growth promoters, and also hormones to increase the supply of milk per cow. The farmers making goats' milk products seem to be more ecologically aware and are not interfering with nature to boost the milk yield artificially, so it is better to choose these dairy products.

Yogurt is beneficial for your health when it contains the culture lactobacillus acidophilus, which is a natural inhabitant of your gut. When yogurts are heat treated, they lose their original culture, so no benefit can be gained from eating them. They are also very acid forming. Fruit yogurt can have a very high sugar content, so it is better to choose a natural bio yogurt and add your own fruit.

Include essential fat in your diet

The important point about fat is that some fats are essential and good for you and some are definitely not. Unfortunately fat has gotten itself a bad name over the years. There have been low-fat diets and no-fat diets, both of which can be dangerous. Because your body cannot make essential fats, the only source is from your diet. Total fat-free diets have resulted in joint stiffness, skin problems, and vaginal dryness.

When considering fats, it is vital to appreciate the difference between those that can contribute to poor health and those that are necessary for good health. Basically, there are two types of fats—saturated and unsaturated.

Saturated fats come from animals (meat, cheese, eggs, etc.) and also from palm kernel oil. These are not essential for your health, and in excess they can cause ill health. They are detrimental to health in two ways:

1. By increasing fat deposits—the more saturated a fat becomes, the harder it is for your body to use it, and so the fat gets deposited and stored unhealthily in the body. Hence the connection between fat intake and hardening of the arteries. The more liquid the saturated fat is at body temperature, the more easily your body uses it, and so there is less chance of it being deposited. The most easily used saturated fat is butter, followed by coconut oil, palm oil, and then fat from beef, lamb, and pork, which is hard at body temperature.

2. By blocking the use of the essential fats—saturated fats interfere with your unsaturated fat metabolism.

Unsaturated fats are a group of fats that include those that are called essential fatty acids, which, as their name implies, are essential for your health. These essential fats are a vital component of every human cell, and your body needs them to insulate your nerve cells, keep your skin and arteries supple, balance your hormones, and keep you warm. These essential fatty acids have been found to relieve benign breast disease, most especially fibrocystic disease, which is also linked with caffeine intake.

They are found in nuts, seeds, oily fish, and vegetables. A handful of nuts or a salad dressing made with a good-quality oil is sufficient for your needs each day. You should also try including in your diet oily fish such as mackerel or sardines.

Unsaturated fats fall into two main groups, monounsaturated and polyunsaturated:

1. Monounsaturated fats (olive oil is high in monounsaturated fats) are so called because they have only one double bond (chemically speaking).
2. Polyunsaturated fats (sunflower oil is high in polyunsaturated fats) can have two or more double bonds.
  Within this group there is a further split into omega 3 fatty acids (the most important of which is alpha-linolenic acid) and omega 6 fatty acids (the most important of which is linolenic acid).
  • Omega 6 oils are found in unrefined safflower, corn, sesame, and sunflower oils.
  • Omega 3 oils are found in fish oils and linseed oil, with varying amounts in pumpkin seeds, walnuts, and dark green vegetables. It is this type of essential fatty acid that is most lacking in our diet. It has been found to enhance immune function, increase metabolic rate and energy levels, and soften the skin.
    Your body makes beneficial prostaglandins (hormone-like regulating substances) from omega 3 oils. These prostaglandins are particularly useful at the

time of menopause, as they help lower blood pressure, decrease inflammation response, and decrease sodium and water retention. They also help keep blood platelet stickiness down, which helps to protect against heart attacks and strokes. A study in 1986 published in the *Journal of the National Cancer Institute* showed that linolenic acid killed human cancer cells in tissue culture without harming the normal cells.

CHOOSING AND USING OILS

Careful choice, storage, and use of oils are essential, as they can easily be damaged. If an oil becomes damaged, oxidation may take place. This leaves the oil open to attack by highly reactive chemical fragments called free radicals. These free radicals have been linked to cancer, coronary heart disease, rheumatoid arthritis, and premature aging. Free radicals speed up the aging process by destroying healthy cells as well as attacking collagen (''cement'' that holds cells together), which is the primary organic constituent of bone, cartilage, and connective tissue. As you get older there is a decrease in collagen, which can cause changes to your skin (wrinkles, prominent veins, slow healing of wounds, vulnerability to bruising), nails (brittleness), eyes (dryness, dark circles under the eyes), gums (bleeding, infection), hair (dullness, split ends, poor growth, hair loss), and mouth (bad breath, mouth ulcers).

Restrict free radical formation by taking these measures:

❑ Choose cold-pressed unrefined vegetable oils or extra-virgin olive oil. Unfortunately most supermarket oils are manufactured and extracted with chemicals and heat, so that the maximum amount of oil is obtained from each batch. This destroys the quality of the oil and the nutritional content. Anti-foaming agents may also have been added to the oils.

❑ Avoid hydrogenated vegetable oils, which are listed in the ingredients of most margarine and also many fast foods, some potato chips, cookies, and crackers. The process of hydrogenation changes the essential unsaturated fats contained in the food into trans fatty acids, which have been linked to an increased rate of heart attack. It is for this reason that I would recommend using butter in moderation or unhydrogenated margarine (obtained from health food shops), rather than ordinary margarine. Although margarine is manufactured from polyunsaturated fats, it is made into a solid form through hydrogenation. The process of hydrogenation makes terrifying reading:

1. Vegetable oil is mixed thoroughly with fine particles of nickel or copper.
2. It is heated to approximately 400°F (200°C) and held at that temperature for six hours.
3. Meanwhile, hydrogen gas is pumped through the mixture at high pressure and the excited hydrogen atoms penetrate the vegetable oil molecules and chemically change them into "trans fats" (trans fatty acids). These are new, complex substances which are not found in nature, except at low levels in some animal fats.
4. The mixture must be kept very hot—if it cools down, the whole production line will get clogged.
5. The mixture is then cooled down to form tiny hard plastic-like beads, known as hydrogenated oil.
6. The beads of hydrogenated oil are mixed with liquid oil and heated up again to a high temperature. When this cools, you have margarine.

(Reproduced with kind permission from *Now You Can Say Goodbye to Hydrogenated Fats* (1994), a leaflet supplied by Whole Earth Foods.)

Because these trans fats are not natural in such high levels and have a plastic-like quality, your body has great difficulty in trying to eliminate or utilize them. Your body is then put under extra pressure simply to deal with a substance that you do not really need to eat.

❑ Do not fry with polyunsaturated fats, as they can become oxidized when heated. Use olive oil or butter for frying.

Monounsaturated olive oil has less chance of creating free radicals, and butter does not because it is saturated. Reduce temperature to minimize oxidation. Keep all fats to a minimum when frying; try to bake or broil instead.

❏ Do not store oil in clear bottles, as light can cause damage.

SUPPLEMENTING ESSENTIAL FATTY ACIDS

As we eat fats, our bodies make them more and more complex. The omega 6 series, linolenic acid, is converted to gamma linolenic acid (GLA) which is found in evening primrose oil. The omega 3 series starting with alpha-linolenic acid is converted into eicospentaenoic acid (EPA), which is found in fish. There are a number of factors that can stop the conversion of linolenic acid into GLA.

As these essential fatty acids are so vital at the time of menopause, it is advisable to supplement them in your diet in the form in which the conversion has already taken place—that is, GLA and EPA—just in case your body is not converting them properly. You can get GLA from evening primrose, borage, black currants, or starflower. Whichever supplement you choose, read the GLA content on the back of the container and aim for a supplement that gives you at least 150mg. of GLA per day. With EPA aim for a supplement that will give you at least 300mg. per day.

Increase the natural fiber in your diet

Fiber in its natural form is helpful in balancing blood sugar levels, but it is known mainly for its action on the bowel and the beneficial effects on problems such as constipation. Fiber binds water and increases the bulk of the stools, so that they are easier to eliminate from the body. This prevents putrefaction of food. If food stays in the bowel too long, it starts to putrefy and ferment (produce gas) inside you, leading to problems of bloating and flatulence, which are common during the menopause. Fiber also aids diges-

---

Recommendations for improving your intake of essential fat

Include:
- Cold-pressed, unrefined vegetable oils such as sesame, sunflower, safflower for salad dressing. Store them in the refrigerator.
- Extra-virgin olive oil for cooking.
- Butter in moderation for spreading or cooking (organic preferably).
- Nuts (almonds, pecans, brazils, etc.) and seeds (sesame, sunflower, pumpkin, etc.).
- Nut butters—made without sugar or palm oil.
- Tahini (creamed sesame seeds) for sauces and dressings.
- Oily fish such as mackerel, sardines, etc.
- Unhydrogenated margarines.

Avoid:
- Commercially produced vegetable oils whose labels do not state that they have been cold-pressed or are extra-virgin.
- Heating oils to high temperatures.
- Storing oils in the light, i.e., in glass bottles on a windowsill.
- Roasting nuts, as it destroys the oils.
- Palm oil, as it is a saturated fat.
- Hydrogenated margarines—i.e. those made with polyunsaturated vegetable oils which have been hydrogenated.

---

tion, increases your feeling of fullness, and removes toxins from your body.

Although there has been a great deal of interest in fiber over the past twenty years, the focus has been on adding bran to a bad diet to increase the fiber content. However, this misses the point. Bran is a refined food, because it is contained in the grains of cereal plants and then stripped

Recommendations for increasing natural fiber in your diet

Include:
- Plenty of fresh fruit and vegetables (cooked and raw).
- Whole grains (brown rice, whole-wheat bread, grain crackers, and pasta), beans, nuts, and seeds. When you eat muesli (containing raw flakes of various grains) it is necessary to soak it beforehand, preferably overnight, to enable the phytates to be broken down, so they do not affect mineral metabolism.

Avoid or reduce:
- Reduce your intake of refined carbohydrates including cake, bread, and cookies containing white flour and sugar.
- Avoid the use of bran by itself and when added or made into breakfast cereals.

away to be sold by itself. Bran contains phytates, which have a binding effect on certain vital nutrients, such as iron, zinc, and magnesium, and this makes these minerals less absorbable. The phytates also bind calcium, making it harder for the body to absorb this mineral, which is so essential for bone health during the menopause.

It makes much more sense to eat the bran in the form that nature intended by eating the grains in their whole state.

Reduce your sodium intake

Sodium is a mineral that is closely associated with your body's ability to balance water retention and blood pressure. The higher the level of blood sodium, the higher the blood pressure. Potassium works with sodium to regulate your water balance and normalize your heart rhythm. The more sodium you consume, the more potassium you need in order to counteract this effect. Low blood sugar, diuretics, and laxatives can all cause potassium loss. In order to achieve a healthy balance you should

• reduce substances that make you lose potassium, such as alcohol, coffee, sugar, diuretics, and laxatives;
• reduce your sodium intake.

Table salt (sodium chloride) is a major source of sodium in the body. It is estimated that in the West our intake is ten to twenty times more than is necessary. Salt is found naturally in all fruits, vegetables, and grains, so we do not really need to add more to our diet. Not only do we add salt to our food during cooking and at the table, but it is abundant in most convenience and prepared foods, including ketchup, salad dressings, burgers, French fries, cookies, pizzas, etc. Even more sodium is put into the body through sodium nitrate, which is the preservative used in cooked meat, and also monosodium glutamate, a flavor enhancer, used extensively in convenience and Chinese food.

Shop wisely

The key to shopping is to buy your food in the most natural state possible. Ask yourself, "What has happened to this food or drink before I buy it?" Try to buy organic produce which has not been sprayed with chemicals, as the pesticides DDT and kepone contain xenoestrogens, estrogen-like compounds that can upset your own delicate female hormone balance. (Although DDT is banned in the United States, it is still used in some developing countries, and can therefore enter the food chain in imported goods.) The farther your food is from its natural state, the harder life is for your body. Refuse to be influenced by all the marketing hype of convenience foods.

Recommendations for reducing your sodium intake

Include:
- More freshly prepared foods, so that you are aware of all the ingredients.
- Low-sodium alternatives such as Morton's Lite. Chemicals are added to table salt to make it flow freely, so if you want salt, choose sea salt.
- Herbs, garlic, ginger, lemon juice, tamari (wheat-free soy sauce) and miso in cooking to add flavor.

Avoid or reduce:
- Reduce your use of salt, added at the table or in cooking.
- Avoid convenience or prepared foods with a high salt content. Read the label carefully.

READ LABELS

Most of us lead busy lives with little time to spare. However, it is worth investing some of your time to have a look at the labels on foods and drinks before you buy them. Once you are familiar with the best brands to buy, shopping for the most healthful foods becomes quick and automatic.

The ingredients on a label are listed in order of content—the first ingredient being present in the highest amount. Labels do not tell us how much of each ingredient is in the food. So one chicken pie may have more chicken than another and we could not tell.

It is best to avoid any ingredients that sound like a chemistry lesson. These are the contents of a brand of apricot dessert: sugar, hydrogenated vegetable oil, gelling agents (E331, E401, E431), emulsifiers (E447, E322), adipic acid, lactose, caseinate, whey powder, flavorings, artificial sweetener (sodium saccharin), colors (E110, E122, E102, E160a). The first question is: where are the apricots? Logically we know that this isn't natural for us to eat.

So generally avoid any products containing E numbers. Some are fine to eat, as they are naturally derived, but the vast majority are not and have known side effects. Without carrying a reference book with us all the time, we cannot know the difference. If the additive in question is a natural one, many food manufacturers now make this clear because it is a selling point. Some products might list natural annatto coloring on the label, for example. This is, in fact, E160b and has no known adverse effect.

E numbers include permitted colors (some natural, some not), preservatives, permitted antioxidants (some natural, e.g. ascorbic acid—vitamin C), emulsifiers and stabilizers, sweeteners, solvents, mineral hydrocarbons, and modified starches.

It is better to avoid all artificial sweeteners. These are chemicals, and the safety of many of them is in doubt. The Center for Science in the Public Interest has called for a ban on the sweeteners acesulfame-K because it is believed to be carcinogenic. Chemical sweeteners are used in a wide variety of foods and drinks, and for the manufacturers they have the advantage of being cheaper than sugar and, in some cases, sweeter. Saccharin, for instance, is 300 times sweeter than sugar. The danger of these sweeteners is not only their individual effects but also the chemical cocktail that results in the body from consuming a number of them in different foods and drinks over a day. Two artificial sweeteners you are likely to encounter in processed foods are described briefly below.

Aspartame Made from two amino acids. Often sold under the brand names NutraSweet and Natrataste. It was developed by chance in 1965. About 180 times sweeter than sucrose. Used in soft drinks, yogurt, chewing gum, ice cream, salads, alcoholic drinks, hot drink mixes, dry mix desserts.

Sodium Saccharin Made from petroleum materials. Discovered by chance in 1937. About 300 times sweeter than sucrose. Used in soft drinks, canned foods, salad dressings, juice pops, confectionery, pharmaceuticals.

Avoid hydrogenated vegetable oils, which can be found in margarine, potato chips, burgers, and cookies. Look for similar products with "vegetable oils" in the list of ingredients.

Avoid whey, which is the yellow-green byproduct of cheese production. It has a vile taste and an awful smell. Because of the increase in cheese consumption, more whey is produced than before. An article in the *Los Angeles Times*, December 4, 1978, stated:

Not only is there more whey, but it is harder to dispose of. Stricter federal and state regulations prohibit dumping raw whey down sewers. Whey is 100 to 200 times stronger a pollutant than residential sewage and most municipal sewerage plants cannot treat it adequately. Disposal in streams is out because whey depletes waterways of oxygen, rendering them incapable of supporting marine life. Even disposal on used land or gravel pits is often unsuitable because of seepage into water supplies. The solution hit upon by both industry and government is to apply high technology and sophisticated marketing techniques and feed the stuff to humans. Whey is increasingly showing up as a cheap substitute ingredient in a wide range of processed foods, from bakery goods and ice cream to soup mixes and beverages.

Be wary of labels that say "no added sugar" as it can mean no added sugar of any kind or no added sucrose. Don't assume that the sugar content is very low because a food bears a "no added sugar" label. In order to make sugar content look less, the manufacturers break down the sugars into various forms, although they all have relatively the same effects on our bodies. Any words ending in -ose are sugars, e.g.:

Fructose—fruit sugar
Glucose—body blood sugar, fast acting
Dextrose—sugar from cornstarch, chemically identical to
    glucose
Lactose—milk sugar

Maltose—sugar made from starch
Sucrose—common table sugar, made from cane or beet
    sugar.

Always take into account the *total* sugar figures provided.

Be careful, too, of foods whose labels claim to have "less" added sugar. For example, a label may say the food contains 25 percent less added sugar and salt. Although there may be a reduction in the sugar and salt added, the product as a whole could have only 15 percent less total sugar and 20 per cent less total salt than the original brand.

Generally, the longer the ingredients list, the more suspicious you should be about the naturalness of the product.

Manufacturers argue that additives, preservatives, and flavorings, etc. are used in such small quantities that they will not have any adverse effects. However, when you take into account all the small amounts in all the different products we eat and drink every day, these small amounts become larger. We are also producing a chemical cocktail inside ourselves and nobody knows how these chemicals will react together.

We all lead busy lives, so just do the best you can as regards the contents of your food. "Everything in moderation" is the best rule to follow. So if you do need to buy convenience or packaged food, find the best brand you can and go for the shortest chemical-looking ingredients list.

Tips for preparation and cooking

❑ With organic carrots and potatoes, you need only to scrub the skins. Do not peel them, as much of the nutrients are concentrated just under the skin.
❑ Lightly cook vegetables in a little water or steam.
❑ Avoid frying where possible. Try broiling or baking.
❑ Choose cookware with care. Avoid the use of all aluminum cookware, as this is a heavy toxic metal that can enter the food through cooking. The same applies to aluminum foil and containers. Avoid any coated cookware, such as non-stick, that is thought to be carcino-

genic. The best cookware materials are cast iron, enamel, glass, and stainless steel.

Shopping list

Variety is the key to enjoying your food and eating for health. There may be foods mentioned below that you have never tried, so experiment and enjoy yourself. Many foods are available in supermarkets; others can be bought from good health food stores, whole food stores or organic farm stores.

Here is a shopping list of foods that are good to include in your diet during the menopause:

FRUIT

Include plenty of fresh fruit, organic if possible; the only organic fruit I can usually get is apples. You may grow other fruits yourself or know someone who does. Use apples, pears, grapes, plums, peaches, nectarines, bananas, berries, cherries, dates (fresh or dried), melons, oranges, tangerines.

Dried fruits make an enjoyable change: raisins, apricots, dates, prunes, figs, apple rings, etc. When buying dried fruit, avoid any that contain the preserving agent sulfur dioxide, which is also used as a bleaching agent in flour. Sulfur dioxide occurs naturally but is produced chemically for commercial use. It is suspected of being a factor in genetic mutations and an irritant of the alimentary food canal. Sulfur dioxide is used most often on dried apricots to keep them a ''nice'' orange color. The package will state whether or not they are free from sulfur dioxide. Those that are free from preservative will look brown but taste fine. Figs and dates are usually free from sulfur dioxide.

Supermarket dried fruits such as mixed fruit, raisins, cranberries, etc., will often have mineral oil added to them. This gives them a shiny appearance and keeps them separate. You should try to avoid this kind of oil, as it can interfere with your absorption of calcium and phosphorus.

As it passes through your body, mineral oil can pick up and excrete the oil-soluble vitamins (A, D, E, K) which you really want to retain. With particular relevance to the menopause, estrogen and the adrenal hormones will also dissolve in the mineral oil and so be taken from your body.

VEGETABLES

Buy organic if you can, and then only scrub the skins instead of peeling whenever possible. You can enjoy carrots, potatoes, cabbage, Brussels sprouts, cauliflower, celery, cucumber, avocado, peppers, broccoli, corn on the cob, beets, asparagus, artichokes, celeriac, garlic, mushrooms, green beans, snow peas, sugar-snap peas, kale, lettuce, onions, parsnips, rutabagas, turnips, radishes, freshly sprouted seeds (alfalfa, mung beansprouts—the most common one), watercress, pumpkins and squash, sweet potatoes and yams.

GRAINS

If your budget limits the amount of organic produce you can buy, put grains at the top of the shopping list. Grains are very small and can absorb more pesticides than other foods, so it is best to buy organic when you can. Include short-grain brown rice, long-grain brown rice, oatmeal, millet, buckwheat, couscous, bulgur wheat, brown basmati rice, barley and popcorn, which can be cooked in a heavy saucepan.

BREAKFAST CEREALS

Shredded Wheat and Puffed Wheat (and store brands of these) are sugar-free. From health food stores you can buy:

- Amaranth Organic Flakes (just wheat and malt),
- Erewhon Crispy Brown Rice Cereal (organically grown whole-grain brown rice),
- Nature's Path Corn Flakes (organic corn, organic wheat syrup, organic barley malt extract, sea salt),

• Pacific Grain Nutty Rice Crunchy Cereal (organic rice, organic corn, malt syrup).

Many different brands of granola and muesli are available in supermarkets and health food stores. Two top-selling brands of granola are Breadshop and Back to Nature. Familia Swiss Muesli and Familia Fruit and Nut Muesli are also very popular.

BREADS

Whole-wheat bread is delicious and wholesome. You may find good bread in your local health food store. Food for Life makes a good brand called Ezekiel Bread, which is frozen and is available nationally. A lot of the supermarket bread contains either sugar or dextrose and/or flour improvers, so read the labels. If the flour improver is ascorbic acid that's OK as it is a form of vitamin C. Pitas make a change, but check the labels for undesirable ingredients. Some supermarkets have a range of specialty breads (olive, tomato breads) using un-treated white flour, which is acceptable. Also look for organic sprouted breads—fruit, multi-grain, and fruity malt loaf. Rye and pumpernickel breads are good too.

CORN TORTILLA SHELLS

These are very useful for stuffing with a kidney bean filling (you can buy canned cooked kidney beans, but remember to check the label, as some have sugar added).

CRACKERS

Ryvita, Wasa and a number of brands sold in health food stores can be added to your shopping list.

FLOUR

There are a number of strong whole-wheat organic flours for bread making. Two good brands are Arrowhead Mills

Whole Grain Pastry Flour and Ancient Quinoa Whole Grain Pastry Flour.

PASTA

There are various whole-wheat pastas available, including those made by De Boles and by Quinoa (Ancient Harvest). For variety, occasionally try supermarkets' fresh pastas, which are made from white flour. If the rest of your food is good, it is fine to use these white pastas moderately. Health food stores sell corn and vegetable pasta, buckwheat noodles, and rice noodles to add variety.

FLAVORINGS

Choose from ginger, herbs (fresh and dried), lemon juice, sea salt, "lite" salt, miso (soybean paste), mustard (check for added sugar, chemicals, etc.), arrowroot or kuzu for thickening gravies and sauces, mayonnaise (Spectrum Naturals makes one without sugar), soy sauce (choose organic where possible, and avoid any brands with monosodium glutamate; good brands are produced by Eden and San-J), ketchup (Westbrae Natural and Muir Glen organic are worth trying), and salad dressings—with no sugar or chemicals; try Cardini's or Newman's, which have good ingredients and are sold in most supermarkets. Other recommended salad dressings include Annie's Naturals, Up Country Naturals, NASOYA, and Spectrum Naturals—all of which offer a full range of types.

NUTS

You can enjoy almonds, pecans, brazil nuts, walnuts, cashews, pistachios, pine nuts (pignolas), and macadamia nuts. They can be eaten as a snack with raisins during the day or used in cooking or salads. Pine nuts added to brown rice during cooking make an enjoyable change.

SEEDS

Try sunflower, sesame, pumpkin, poppy, and caraway seeds. These can be added to salads or cooked vegetable dishes or put in with rice when cooking.

SEED AND NUT BUTTERS

Excellent organic peanut butters are available; try Woodstock Old Fashioned and Polaner Natural Smooth. Arrowhead Certified Organic produces both peanut and cashew butters. Marantha offers Roasted Sunflower and Organic Almond butters. Tahini (creamed sesame seeds) can be used in salad dressings and is also used in making hummus (a Greek dip made from chickpeas which is available in supermarkets). Two brands to look for are Woodstock and Joyva. When buying nut butters, try to avoid those that contain palm oil, as it is a saturated fat.

SWEETENERS

It is better to rely on the natural sweetness of foods themselves. If you are making a cake, try baking a carrot and raisin or banana cake. Cook with eating apples for apple pies, and you will find you do not need to add any sweetener, but you could add raisins for extra sweetness if needed. Date slice is wonderful because dates are naturally sweet (see the recipe on page 253).

As your taste buds grow accustomed to doing without the very powerful taste of refined sugar you will come to appreciate the sweetness of vegetables and fruits more.

Try maple syrup, concentrated apple juice, date syrup, honey (use sparingly, and avoid those that are "blended" or the "produce of more than one country" as they are often heated to temperatures as high as 160°F [71°C], which destroys their goodness).

If the label says "flavored," in the case of "maple-flavored" syrup, beware: it is not the real thing and will contain sugar and chemical flavoring.

BEANS/LEGUMES

When I first started eating legumes, or pulses, I used to go to my local health food store and stare at the shelves. The beans were in plastic bags with a labeled name and I had no idea what to do with them. With the help of good cookbooks and advice from my health food store, I soon found they were easy to cook with and versatile. As with anything new it is just a case of getting used to them.

Try experimenting with aduki beans, black-eyed peas, chickpeas (used in hummus), kidney beans, navy beans (used in baked beans), lentils (brown and red—wonderful for soups, vegetarian stews, and vegetarian spaghetti bolognese), split peas, lima beans, mung beans (known as beansprouts when sprouted), and soybeans (also used for making tofu, soy sauce, and miso).

MEAT

Meat contains the most saturated fat, so should be kept to a minimum. Of all meat, poultry is the most healthful choice. Some supermarkets sell organic or free-range or corn-fed meat. By not eating meat, we are avoiding not only the saturated fat but also the growth hormones, antibiotics, and other chemicals given to many animals reared for human consumption. On occasions when you may want to eat meat, see if you can get "naturally reared" products.

FISH

You can choose oily fish—mackerel, tuna, fresh salmon, canned salmon (eat the bones), sardines—and most other fish such as cod, flounder, trout, etc.

EGGS

Buy free-range eggs, and if possible buy those eggs labeled, "from hens fed on food free from antibiotics, hormones, and artificial growth promoters" (or words to that effect).

"Free-range" just implies that the hens have a certain amount of freedom as compared to hens kept in cages—they can still be fed on "junk." Our own hormones are going through enough of a balancing act as it is without adding in hormones from outside or artificial growth promoters.

SOY

If you are animal-milk intolerant and find that it causes skin problems or sinus trouble, soy milk is a helpful alternative. Buy organic where possible and make sure the milk is sugar-free. Among the many good brands are Vitasoy, Westbrae, Westsoy, and Health Valley. Most are available with plain, vanilla, and chocolate flavors and in regular and low-fat forms.

Soy milk can be used in cooking in the same way as cows' milk. In cooking you cannot taste the difference between cows' milk and soy milk. Soy can also be used in the form of tofu, which is soybean curd made by adding a curdling agent to soy milk. Tofu can be used in stir-fries, soups, and also desserts. Miso, too, is made from soybeans, combined with rice or barley. A mold culture is added, and the mixture is left to ferment for one to three years. This paste can be added to soups or casseroles.

Soy sauce (shoyu) is made from fermented soybeans and is also sold as tamari, which is wheat-free soy sauce. When you buy soy sauce, make sure it contains just the natural ingredients—soybeans, wheat, water, and salt—and not sugar or MSG (monosodium glutamate).

Tempeh is another type of soybean product, made from fermenting beans and pressing them into a block. Tempeh has a strong taste and can be fried or used in soups.

Soy contains two flavonoid compounds, genistein and daidzein, which have mild estrogenic activity. Japanese women have minimal menopausal problems, and this may be due to the large amount of soy they eat. Soy has also been found to lower cholesterol and help prevent cancer.[1]

RICE DRINKS

Other alternatives to animals' milk are rice drinks. They can be used on cereals, in cooking, and as a drink (hot or cold). The rice milk made by Imagine Foods, called Rice Dream, contains filtered water, organically grown brown rice, safflower oil, and sea salt. Another well-known brand is Pacific Rice.

OAT MILK

This is another alternative to cows' milk and is a mixture of oats, oil, and water (one brand to look for is Westbrae Natural Oat Plus).

DAIRY PRODUCE

Use organic dairy produce where possible. If you have a milk allergy, try sheep's or goats' milk or a non-animal drink like soya or rice. Buy live yogurt containing the culture lactobacillus acidophilus—organic if possible. If you like fruit yogurt, use the live yogurt and add your own fruit. Frozen yogurt makes a refreshing summer dessert; use a regular recipe and substitute maple syrup or honey for the sugar.

OIL/FAT

Use butter (organic if possible) and unhydrogenated margarines (Spectrum Naturals and Sheda's Willow Run margarine, both unhydrogenated, can be obtained from health food stores). Look for cold-pressed, unrefined vegetable oils like sesame, sunflower, safflower. Buy extra-virgin olive oil for light cooking.

DRINKS

As a substitute for coffee, try Caro and Caro Extra, Bambu, and Yannoh, which are grain ''coffees'' and contain various combinations of ingredients such as barley, rye, chicory, and acorns. Instead of tea, try herb teas, fruit teas, decaffeinated tea (such as Great Eastern Sun organically grown teas), Japanese twig (bancha) tea.

When you use herb (not fruit) teas on a regular basis, remember that herbs have specific effects, so it is better to use a variety of herbs than to stick to one kind. For example, peppermint tea is very good for aiding digestion, so is excellent to drink after a meal. Chamomile tea is relaxing and is often drunk at the end of the day to help insomnia. It also has an anti-inflammatory action which is useful in the digestive system for easing diverticulitis as well as general colon problems. (Reputable manufacturers of teas include Celestial Seasonings, Heath and Heather, and Yogi Tea.)

SOFT DRINKS

Use real unsweetened fruit juice. If a carton or bottle has "fruit drink" on the label, you know that something else has been added. A recent analysis of fruit drinks showed that many had only 5 percent fruit, while the rest of the drink was made up of water, sugar, and additives. Liven up fruit juice with sparkling mineral water if you like. Or try the sparkling apple juices, such as Martinelli and After the Fall cider. The latter company makes soft drinks in a wide range of flavors, as do R. W. Knudson Family and Journy.

CONVENIENCE FOODS

Baked beans

Most of the baked beans in the supermarkets will contain a fair amount of sugar. If the label states "sugar-free," they may well have an artificial sweetener added, instead, so check the ingredients list carefully. Health Valley Fat-Free Honey Baked Beans are a nutritious alternative to the artificially sweetened brands.

Soups

In supermarkets it is difficult to find soups that do not contain sugar, artificial sweeteners, or chemicals. However, in health food stores you can find a good range, including those made by Health Valley, Westbrae (their Natural Soups of the World), and Shari's Bistro Organic. Health Valley offers Healthy Soup in a Cup, and Image Natural produces soup in cartons.

Ready made meals

Even with the best intentions in the world, it may sometimes be necessary to have a supply of quick, ready made, wholesome food. For a quick meal, I would tend to use pasta and make a sauce with a good-quality canned tomato sauce and serve this with a salad. Or just have plain broiled fish with vegetables and/or rice. Muir Glen Organic, Seeds of Change, and Millina's Finest all make spaghetti sauces which are useful if time is really short. Most of the ready made sauces in the supermarkets contain sugar, so again it's worth reading the labels for a while, until you are familiar with the brands that are best for you. There are some reasonable frozen meals available, but keep these for emergencies and cook from fresh where possible.

Snacks and cookies

Fresh fruit, dried fruit, nuts and mixed nuts, and raisins are all good and tasty to use as a snack at any time. You can get good-quality potato chips and tortilla (corn) chips from health food stores and supermarkets. Some manufacturers use sea salt in these products. With potato and tortilla chips, check whether the oil is hydrogenated. If it is, buy another brand. Ryvita and rice cakes (there are many flavors) are fine to eat.

Health food stores offer an amazing variety of nutritious cookies and fruit bars, including some that are made without wheat. (If you suffer from bloating or digestive problems, you may have a wheat allergy, which should be checked by a good nutritional therapist.) Some tempting varieties are made by 100% Natural Organic Lady J Cookies; sweetened with fruit juice, they include Peanut Butter, Chocolate Chunk, and Wheat-free, Sugar-free Date. Westbrae makes Natural Ginger Snaps Rice Malt Cookies, which are made with organic whole wheat and are sugar-free. The ever-popular graham cracker has been enhanced by Hain Pure Foods, who offer it in three varieties: Honey, Cinnamon, and French Vanilla. Fig bars, too, come in new guises. Barbara's Fig Bars, which are sweetened with fruit juice, are available in Blueberry and Raspberry pairings, as well as in the Traditional (fig only) and Wheat-free, Fat-free forms. In a pun on the name of the best-known brand, Paul Newman offers his own organic Fig Newmans.

In looking for alternatives to ordinary sweet snacks, do not substitute diabetic ones, which contain sorbitol. Sorbitol is a sugar alcohol which occurs naturally in some fruits and is metabolized in our bodies. For commercial use, it is synthesized chemically from glucose. Diabetics are advised to eat foods containing only a certain amount of sorbitol per day because it can have adverse side effects such as flatulence, diarrhea, and bloating. It does not raise the blood level significantly, as would sugar or pure glucose, but it is chemically processed, not natural, and should be avoided.

Jams and jellies

There are some very good-quality sugar-free jams and jellies available, from supermarkets as well as health food stores. Be wary, though: if you see a supermarket jam marked "sugar-free," check the label for artificial sweeteners. The jam should be made solely from real fruit.

Note the color also. It has been known for some jam-making companies to extract the color from the fruit (e.g. strawberries) during the jam making and then at the end add in artificial colors. The "real" jams may not look quite as bright as these, but they taste delicious, and after all, you're eating them for the taste and quality, not the color.

Officially the word "jam" means a preserve, which implies that it contains sugar to act as a preservative; so the natural sugar-free jams are usually called "spreads." They contain only real fruit and a setting agent, such as pectin from limes. The choice of flavors, in both jams and jellies, is quite amazing, including raspberry, blackberry, wild blueberry, and apricot (one of the most successful). Grape jelly, made from both white and Concord grapes, is readily available. Brands of jelly and jam to look for include Polaner All Fruit, Cascadian Farm Organic, and St. Dalfours, imported from France. Also worth trying are Woodstock Orchard's Apple Spread and Lekvar Prune Butter.

Desserts

As you steer away from pre-packaged foods, it becomes more necessary to make your own desserts. For quickness, you can rely on fresh fruit, either whole or in a fruit salad or yogurt. Baked eating apples are easy to prepare with a stuffing of raisins. Stewed fruit or compotes can also be made.

At health food stores you can get sugar-free puddings in flavors such as lemon, butterscotch, and banana. Brands include Imagine and Luppe. Supermarkets now have a good range of canned fruit that is packed in fruit juice rather than syrup. Fresh fruit is always preferable, but canned fruit could be added to a fresh fruit compote for variety.

Seaweed/sea vegetables

The name "seaweed" is somewhat off-putting and so I prefer to use the term "sea vegetables," which is what these plants are. In the United States, packages of dried sea vegetables are sold in health food shops. They are low in calories and fat-free and have a very good mineral content, including the trace minerals zinc, manganese, chromium, selenium, and cobalt and the macro minerals calcium, magnesium, iron, and iodine. A valid criticism has been that because they are obviously harvested from the sea, they could be laden with heavy toxic metals such as lead, cadmium, and mercury. However, if you buy from a reputable company such as Great Eastern Sun, producers of Emerald Cove brand, you can be assured that the sea vegetables are harvested in clear water away from known areas of pollution where the sea water is regularly tested. After harvesting, the sea vegetables are also tested independently for heavy metal contamination. Good seaweeds to try are of kelp, wakame, nori, and hijiki.

Bon appetit!

CHAPTER 6

Natural alternatives to HRT

As I have said, this book is all about choices. Also, as you will have gathered, I am very much opposed to the idea that hormone replacement therapy should be the first thing women think about when they begin to experience menopausal symptoms. In many cases I don't feel that the actual cause of these symptoms is the menopause itself—though it may exacerbate and act as a kind of catalyst for problems that are already there. Our diets, our lifestyles, our lack of essential nutrients may well be exposed by this particular event. For while hot flashes and vaginal dryness may be specific to the menopause, other symptoms, such as mood swings, painful breasts, and water retention, are often associated with premenstrual problems also. Once a woman reaches a certain age it's very easy to label all her symptoms "menopausal." Many of these symptoms are less to do with a shortage of hormones and much more to do with an imbalance. It is restoring the balance, instead of pumping ourselves full of outside hormones, that is the key. There are numerous different ways we can do this without resorting to powerful drugs. Besides getting our nutrition right, we can use natural therapies to combat particular problems and improve our overall health. And these therapies can bring us to a fuller understanding of the way our bodies work. Once this is grasped, it will become clear that the menopause is not a medical condition but a natural event that our bodies, given the chance, should cope with perfectly happily.

Which therapy should you choose? Below I give a brief description of each therapy. Then I suggest how each one can help your specific symptoms. All these therapies are complementary to orthodox Western medicine. And different complementary therapies can be used together. The main criticism of this approach is that if you use more than one therapy at the same time, you may not know which one made the difference to your health. But does this matter? You are not conducting a controlled experiment—you just want to feel well. Some practitioners are quite protective and are not happy if you see somebody else from another discipline at the same time as seeing them. I personally feel it can be an advantage. Because we are all individuals, some therapies may work better than others for you.

What are the choices?

NUTRITIONAL THERAPY

Most of us don't realize it, but food is, and should be regarded as, a powerful medicine which has a huge impact on the biochemical processes of the body. Nutritional therapy is not just about eating well. It is also about correcting any vitamin or mineral deficiencies. You need to eat a good variety of food and not restrict yourself to a small range, so as to give yourself the best chance of getting all the nutrients you need. You then need to look at any particular symptoms to see if there any areas that may require supplementation. It's important to remember that supplements are just that—extra—and not a substitute for healthy food and a well-balanced diet.

One of the most dramatic examples by recent scientific research is the effect of foods containing natural substances known as phytoestrogens on female hormones. High levels of phytoestrogens are found in foods such as soy. Scientists are fascinated by phytoestrogens because they now believe these naturally occurring weak estrogens may hold the key to curing and preventing breast cancer, more of which later. But their research, reported in the *British Medical Journal*, has also shown that supplementing the diet of postmenopausal women with soy and other foods containing phytoestrogens (linseed oil and red clover sprouts) reduced their amount of FSH (the hormone that rises at the menopause) to premenopausal levels—putting the clock back naturally.[1] The women's diet was supplemented with soy flour (10g daily), linseed oil (25g daily) and red clover sprouts (10g daily), and these foods made up only 10 percent of their total diet during this experiment, very little indeed. Yet the effect of these phytoestrogens was strong enough to have a rapid and noticeable effect on the cells of the vagina, reducing vaginal dryness and irritation. These effects were detectable in just a few weeks and lasted for two months after the foods had been stopped, demonstrating that the consumption of phytoestrogens is crucial to fending off menopausal symptoms and explaining why Japanese and other Oriental women, whose diet is loaded with soy, rarely complain about hot flashes or other menopausal symptoms. Other sources of phytoestrogens include fennel, celery, parsley, rhubarb, and hops.

Another example of the power of food is the effect of an extract from rice called gamma-oryzanol, which has been found to be effective in relieving both menopausal and menstrual imbalances.[2] Supplementing your diet with 20mg per day of gamma-oryzanol helps with hot flashes and a number of other symptoms. It can be taken as capsules, available from health food stores.

The vitamins and minerals we require for our bodies to function work in harmony, and most of them are dependent on each other in order to act efficiently. The best way to structure a supplement program for yourself is to take a good all-around multivitamin and mineral supplement designed for the menopause, including supplies of magnesium, calcium, and boron. Good brands are New Chapter, New Spirit Naturals, Vita Balance 2000, and Rainbow Light. You should also take linseed oil in capsule form, as this has also been shown to help with calcium balance.[3] You can then add in any supplements that relate specifically to your symptoms. The basic multivitamin and mineral supplement forms the foundation of the program; others then are included, depending on the particular symptoms you experience.

When it comes to buying mineral or vitamin supplements, you get what you pay for. I would recommend buying capsules instead of tablets. Capsules tend to be filled only with active ingredients. Tablets can include a variety of fillers, binders, and bulking agents. Mineral supplements such as calcium should be in the form of citrates, ascorbates, or polynicotinates, which are more easily absorbed by the body. Chlorides, sulfates, carbonates, and oxides should be avoided, since they are not so easily assimilated, and mineral supplements in this form may pass through the body without being absorbed. So it's important to read the labels. The other way minerals are made more digestible is by chelation (pronounced "keylation"). Chelated minerals allow three to ten times' greater assimilation than the non-chelated ones.

It could be argued that HRT is a supplement, just as vitamins and minerals are, and that by taking it we are only supplying what is lacking. There is, however, a major difference between nutritional supplements and HRT. Hormones are chemical compounds produced internally by the body itself. HRT, a powerful drug, contains hormones synthesized from an external source and then introduced into the body. Vitamins, on the other hand, are chemical compounds that cannot be synthesized by the body. Vitamins and minerals can be obtained only from foods and supplements and generally cannot be produced internally.

From the food we eat and the nutrients that food gives us, our bodies are able to produce whatever hormones we need. Nutritional or food supplements are the building blocks providing those same nutrients, albeit in a more concentrated form than we may require, in order for our bodies to function at optimum health. Supplements are, in crude terms, a concentrated form of food and as such are completely natural.

If we are not in good health or our hormones are out of balance, our wisest course is to go back to basics and obtain the right nutrients (food and/or food supplements). This returns us to optimum health, allowing our own bodies to produce the correct level of hormones again and get them back in balance.

HERBS

As with food supplements herbs can be used to obtain optimum health so that your body can balance your hormones, heal itself, and help to prevent illness and disease from getting a hold. Herbal medicine is the oldest form of medicine, and herbs have been used for healing in all cultures and in all times. Herbs are, in fact, the foundation of numerous pharmaceutical drugs. Aspirin is based on an extract from willow, originally used for pain relief by Native Americans, and steroids have been derived from wild yam. Up to 70 percent of drugs in use today have their origins in plants. But Western pharmaceutical practice is to use the active ingredient of the plant or herb in a pure form of a determined strength and quantity as the basis for the drug. When a plant or herb is used in its whole form, as in herbal medicine, the side effects are absent or minimal. In earlier times, for example, the foxglove plant (*Digitalis purpurea*) was used for heart problems. In modern times, scientists have been able to isolate the main active ingredient of the foxglove (digoxin). However, if only the active ingredient is used, in a drug form, there is the real risk of side effects. If the whole plant is used, the active ingredient interacts with all the other constituents of the plant, which naturally includes "buffer" ingredients that counteract the side effects. Herbalists believe this is the proper way to use the healing powers of herbs and plants.

The best way to use herbs is to choose those that have a balancing effect on your hormones without directly supplying one hormone or another. These balancing agents are called adaptogens. Adaptogenic herbs allow the body to restore itself naturally without causing an imbalance in any hormone or body system. These herbs tone and strengthen the whole of the reproductive system. Examples include chasteberry (vitex), black cohosh, blue cohosh, and false unicorn root. Below I have given a guide for the general use of these and other herbs at the menopause. If you have specific symptoms such as fibroids, etc., it would be worth consulting a good herbalist or a health professional with experience in using herbs, because some can have a direct hormone-like action and are used in specific conditions while best avoided for others.

For general use, it is better to have a number of herbs mixed together. Some herbs work better for some women than others do, so if you have an appropriate "menopause" mix you can be sure of having a good balance.

The easiest and most effective way of taking herbs is in tincture form (approximately 1 teaspoon [5ml] three times daily in a little water). Try to get tinctures made from organically grown herbs. In the liquid form the herbs are already dissolved; hence they are available faster and their action is quicker. In the dry form, the tablets or capsules have to be digested, and the benefit of the herbs is only as good as your digestive and absorption processes. You will find that as the herbs rebalance your hormones you can reduce the dose, bringing it down to 2.5ml. (½ teaspoon) three times a day, for example, and eventually discontinuing the herbs altogether. Herbs are not like drugs. If drugs are stopped, the symptoms can return, and you are back where you started. The herbs stop the symptoms. But they are also addressing the cause at the same time, so the symptoms are being alleviated because the body is becoming more balanced.

HOMEOPATHY

The word "homeopathy" comes from the Greek words *omio*, meaning "same" and *pathos*, meaning "suffering." It is a treatment of "like with like" so that the person complaining of certain symptoms is given a homeopathic remedy that produces the same symptoms. Homeopathy was founded by Samuel Hahnemann, a German doctor, and is an extremely safe form of medicine which works on the principle of helping the body to fight its own battles by prescribing in minute amounts. It is in direct contrast to allopathic medicine (most Western medicine), which treats symptoms by trying to create the opposite effect from which the person is complaining. If a person is feeling very stressed and anxious and has palpitations, for instance, the practitioner would prescribe a homeopathic remedy that in a healthy person would actually create that same set of symptoms, thereby encouraging the body's own healing mechanisms. Modern conventional medicine, on the other hand, would prescribe drugs such as tranquilizers and beta blockers to create calmness.

In homeopathy, different people may be prescribed different remedies for the same illness. Homeopaths take a very detailed history of the individual and look not only at the symptoms the person is suffering from now but also at such things as their likes and dislikes, any food cravings, whether they are a hot or cold person, their personality characteristics, and their physical type. The remedy prescribed is then called a "constitutional remedy" and is individual to that person.

The remedies listed below are "symptomatic," but if you are experiencing symptoms of long standing which are not improving, it would be better to seek help from a qualified homeopath who will be able to treat you constitutionally.

A number of remedies are recommended for the menopause; these can be chosen depending on the kind and severity of symptoms you are experiencing. (If you don't find the one you need in your health food store, ask them to order it for you.) These remedies are to be taken every twelve hours for up to seven days with a potency of 30C. (This is a measure of the concentration of a remedy. The higher the number, the more potent the remedy.)

Sepia is one of the main remedies for the menopause. It is useful for heavy periods, hot flashes, and headaches, and also if you are easily depressed and irritable.

Lachesis is for flooding during periods, irritability, forgetfulness, hot flashes, and a headache on waking.

Pulsatilla is especially suited to those who have fair hair and who cry easily.

Kali carb is useful if the symptoms are worse in the middle of the night and also where there is loss of appetite.

Graphites is beneficial for those women who have scanty periods, weight gain, and hot flashes.

Sanguinaria is useful for tender breasts and heavy periods.

Conium is helpful where there is a lack of sex drive.

AROMATHERAPY

Aromatherapy is the use of essential plant oils for healing. The oils themselves have been popular for centuries. Egyptians used frankincense for embalming, and Cleopatra was reputed to have seduced Mark Antony by wearing jasmine oil—perhaps one to try for an evening in at home! Hippocrates, ''the father of medicine,'' stated that ''the way to good health is to take an aromatic bath and fragrant massage every day.'' During the two world wars, clove, thyme, and chamomile oil were used as substitutes for scarce disinfectants.

The term ''aromatherapy'' was used in the thirties by the French chemist René Gatefosse. While working in a laboratory, he burned his hand; to ease the pain, he plunged it into a nearby bowl of lavender oil. The burn healed quickly with little scarring. Impressed by this, he began to investigate the medicinal powers of pure essential oils. Essential oils are found in the stem, flowers, leaves, bark, seeds, or peel of aromatic plants. Once extracted, these become more concentrated and potent. Each essential oil has its own specific properties and works on two levels: through our sense of smell and by being absorbed into the bloodstream via the skin and lungs, where it has a therapeutic effect on organs, glands, and tissue. The oils are volatile, so must be kept in dark glass bottles out of the sun at a cool temperature. If the essential oil is to come into contact with your skin it must be blended in a carrier oil, such as almond oil (exceptions are lavender oil and tea tree oil) or diluted in water. Drops of essential oil can be used directly in the bath.

There are a number of ways of using essential oils.

Massage

Massage is very popular as a way of targeting problem areas or your whole body. You can have a bath or shower first so that the oil is better absorbed. Do not use it on broken or infected skin. Use 5 drops of essential oil to 10ml. (2 teaspoons) of carrier oil. If you have sensitive skin, you can use jojoba oil as a carrier oil.

Bath or shower

With a bath, add the essential oil just before you step into the bath so that the oil is strong. Don't have the water too hot, or the oil will disperse quickly. Make sure the room is warm, soak for ten to fifteen minutes, and inhale the steam while you soak. Use 5 drops of essential oil directly into a full bath.

For a shower, stay under the spray and massage the oil using a mitt or sponge. Use 5 drops of essential oil to 10ml. (2 teaspoons) of carrier oil.

Footbath

Put 4 drops of essential oil directly into a bowl of warm water, and soak your feet for fifteen to twenty minutes.

Inhalation

Fill a basin with hot water, add 2 to 3 drops of essential oil directly into the water, and make a tent over your head with a towel so that none of the aromatic steam escapes. Breathe deeply for five minutes, keeping your eyes closed.

Other ways to inhale:

- Place a few drops on a tissue or pillow
- Add a few drops to a bowl of water, and place the bowl near a radiator so the oil vaporizes
- Add 8 drops of oil to 300ml. (1¼ cups) of water to use as a room spray

- Use scented lightbulb rings, essential oil burners, and steam vaporizers.

The most suitable oils for the menopause are chamomile, geranium, rose, jasmine, neroli, ylang-ylang, bergamot, sandalwood, and clary sage.

ACUPUNCTURE

This ancient system of Chinese medicine dates back some 2,000 years and is based on the concept of *Qi* (pronounced "chee"), which is the body's energy. Having the right balance of *Qi* in the various channels or meridians of the body is the fundamental principle of traditional Chinese medicine. The acupuncturist aims to influence this flow of *Qi* to balance the physical and mental aspects of a person. It has been remarkably successful in treating severe menstrual or menopausal problems. Acupuncture can be used with the other complementary medicine therapies to correct hormone and energy imbalances during the menopause. This is obviously not a self-help system, so you need to see a qualified acupuncturist. Some medical doctors also practice acupuncture.

Natural alternatives to HRT for menopausal symptoms

There are several common menopausal symptoms. You might suffer just one of them—or all of them at different times. Here's how you can use the natural alternatives outlined above to cope with specific problems.

ANXIETY AND IRRITABILITY

Make sure that you keep your blood sugar level in balance. This is explained in the chapter on nutrition (see page 45). It is important that you eliminate from your diet "stimulants" such as tea, coffee, and sugar, which give a quick rise in blood sugar followed by a rapid drop. As your blood sugar levels drop, your body will release the hormone adrenaline to try to correct this imbalance. Adrenaline is the hormone that is also released when you are under stress, so you will experience those same feelings of anxiety and tension—even when there is no external stress at all. For the same reason, you should eat little and often. If you go more than three hours without food, adrenaline will be released into the system again.

Nutritional therapy

Magnesium is classed as "nature's tranquilizer," so it is worth adding to your diet in the form of a supplement. The B vitamins are well known for their ability to help with stress, so these should also be included. Take:

Magnesium—300mg per day
Vitamin B complex containing 100mg of each B vitamin—once per day.

Herbs

In herbal medicine, herbs that help us to feel calm are called nervines. They act on the nervous system to relieve anxiety, tension, and irritability. One of the best-known herbs for anxiety and tension is valerian. It is effective when combined with skullcap, which also relaxes the nervous system and at the same time can renew a flagging nervous system. Skullcap has been used for premenstrual tension, too, and since this is the time of the month when we tend to feel most irritable, it is a good herb to choose.

Ginseng is good for anxiety and tension. Panax (Korean or Chinese) ginseng is often used as a tonic, since it helps the adrenal glands function. Studies have shown that the use of panax ginseng can help us withstand the effects of many different stressful situations and increase our mental alertness. It can boost vitality and physical performance. Siberian ginseng also helps in stressful situations and has a more subtle effect than panax ginseng. Both ginsengs are classed herbally as adaptogens and have a normalizing, balancing effect on the body.

Aromatherapy

Clary sage is wonderful for lifting your mood and seems to be particularly effective blended with geranium. Put 7 drops of clary sage and 7 drops of geranium in a carrier oil. Use in your bath or as a massage.

BREAST TENDERNESS/LUMPY BREASTS

Up to 70 percent of women have fibrocystic breasts—tender, swollen breasts and swollen lumps that fluctuate with the menstrual cycle and may become more obvious and painful in the very early stages of the menopause. Excess estrogen may be the cause of this rather frightening condition, which is not however, thought to have any link to breast cancer. Avoid drinks that contain methylxanthines (coffee, tea, chocolate, cola, and even decaffeinated coffee), as these have been shown to cause breast lumps.[4] If you eat red meat or poultry, try to choose organic meat from animals that have not been raised on synthetic hormones. Try to buy organic milk, too, as ordinary milk contains female hormones which the cows have been given to increase their milk production. We also get excess hormones from our tap water, which contains residues from the Pill and HRT as well as xenoestrogens from petrochemical companies depositing their waste in rivers.

Nutritional therapy

A diet high in saturated fat is known to stimulate estrogen overproduction, so a diet free of animal products, except fish, could help.[5] Increase your intake of oily fish and nuts or seeds or supplement with fish oils or linseed oil. Vitamin E acts as an antioxidant, so may help protect your breasts against excess estrogen. It also has anti-inflammatory and hormone-regulating actions. Because vitamin E can be contraindicated with raised blood pressure, check with your health professional before taking it if you are prone to high blood pressure.

Adding lactobacillus acidophilus as a supplement seems to help, because it lowers the level of the enzymes that reabsorb the "old" estrogen. Also, if there is a deficiency in the B vitamins, the liver cannot inactivate "old" estrogens, and vitamin B6 alone has been shown to raise progesterone levels which would keep the estrogen more in balance.[6] Take:

Vitamin E—400–1000ius per day
Linseed oil capsules—1000mg per day
Acidophilus—one capsule morning and night
Vitamin B complex—50mg twice per day

There is a link between fibrocystic breast disease and constipation, for which I have given some suggested remedies below. One study in the British medical journal *The Lancet* in 1981 showed that women who had fewer than three bowel movements per week had a 4.5 times greater chance of having breast problems than women who had a bowel movement at least once a day.[7] This makes sense, because if we are not eliminating all the waste and toxic products from our bodies effectively, we can literally be storing up trouble. It has been suggested that certain microorganisms in bowel matter are capable of actually recycling old estrogen that our bodies should actually be eliminating. Because it is thought that breast problems are due to excess estrogen, it is vital that we eliminate all our "used" estrogens. Another study showed that the dietary fiber we eat in the form of grains and vegetables reduces estrogen levels and seems to work by "shielding" estrogens which are excreted in the bile from being reabsorbed back into the blood. Women who ate a vegetarian diet excreted three times more "old," detoxified estrogens than women who also ate meat. The meat eaters also reabsorbed more estrogens.

Herbs

Lumpy or tender breasts may be a sign that estrogen is not being processed efficiently by the liver. Some beneficial herbs for the liver may help.

Dandelion helps to cleanse the liver, the major organ of detoxification, which also gets rid of accumulated ''old'' female hormones. If the liver is functioning effectively, this prevents excess estrogen from building up and increasing the risk of breast growths and other cell changes.

Milk thistle is also an excellent herb for the liver, and a number of studies have shown that its use can result in an increase of new liver cells to replace old damaged ones.[8] Silymarin is the collective name for the substances found in milk thistle which have this beneficial effect.

Vitex can be used for breast tenderness because of its ability to normalize the female hormones. Using this herb can help to correct any imbalances of excess estrogen.

Wild yam can also be used to balance estrogen.

CONSTIPATION

It is important that your bowels be working properly. The bowels' function is to get rid of everything that your body doesn't want or need, so if you are not eliminating properly, toxins and poisons can be reabsorbed into your system. It is also important because you need to eliminate ''old'' hormones, especially estrogen, from your body. Make sure you are facilitating this process by eating a good supply of fruits and vegetables.

Nutritional therapy

Take:

Vitamin C—try 3,000mg per day and increase by 500mg at a time until your stools are manageable, soft, and comfortable,

Linseed oil capsules—1000mg twice per day.

Herbs

Herbs can be very useful in this area. Normal laxatives work by stimulating or increasing the number of bowel movements or by encouraging a softer or bulkier stool. Unfortunately they do not address the cause of the problem, such as lack of fiber, and people can become dependent on them. The more these laxatives are used, the less the body has to do for itself, and ultimately the bowel can lose its tone and muscle action, and then the person cannot do without the laxatives. Herbs work in two ways: first to create a healthy and frequent bowel movement and then to tone the bowel to help its own natural function. A number of gentle herbs are useful for constipation; these include butternut, blue flag, and physillium. Good herbal companies will have available readymade capsules of a number of gentle bowel-toning herbs and they will also have capsules or powder to use for a bowel cleanse to help detoxify the colon.

FATIGUE AND LACK OF ENERGY

First check that your iron and thyroid levels are correct. Your doctor can do this. If the levels are all right, again look at your blood sugar balance. Are you having regular cups of coffee or tea during the day which are actually making you feel more tired? Do you need another one to keep yourself going? Are you tired because you are not sleeping well due to night sweats or because of too much tea or coffee? A patient of mine who went to her doctor because she was lacking in energy all through the day was told that she had TATT (tired all the time). She knew that already; what she wanted to know was why and what she could do about it.

Nutritional therapy

If your iron and thyroid checks are fine, try supplementing with co-enzyme Q10, which has been shown to increase energy production in our cells. Co-enzyme Q10 is a substance that is present in all human tissues and organs. It is a vital catalyst in the provision of energy for all human cells. The consequence of a deficiency of co-enzyme Q10 is a reduction in energy and slowing down of life-giving processes. A good balanced diet should contain all the Q10 we need, but unfortunately as we age, our ability to produce Q10 from our diet decreases and we may need a supplement. Take:

Co-enzyme Q10—20–50mg per day
Vitamin E—100ius per day
Vitamin B complex containing 100 mg of each B vitamin—once per day.

Herbs

Either of the ginsengs recommended for anxiety and irritability (see page 95) can help boost your energy and vitality.

Although it is sometimes necessary for us to keep our energy levels going because we have something to finish or we just haven't time to rest, it is not good to do this with stimulants such as tea or coffee. It creates a vicious circle of needing something more often. The same thing can actually happen with some herbs, too. It is all right to use the ginseng to help increase your energy levels, but you need to look at your overall nutrition and health also.

HEADACHES/MIGRAINES

There is a difference between a headache and a migraine headache. Headaches are painful but are not usually accompanied by other symptoms. Headaches can be due to tension or bad posture, perhaps while sitting in one position for too long. These can be relieved with a hot bath with essential oils or an aromatherapy massage. Good oils to use are melissa and lavender. Lavender essential oil can be rubbed into the temples, directly onto the skin, without first being put in a carrier oil.

Migraine headaches, however, usually follow a pattern of symptoms, and these can be different for different people, depending on the type of migraine they get. Some sufferers experience warning symptoms (aura) before the pain starts; these can include blurring and changes in vision, yawning and fatigue, and numbness on one side of the body. The pain itself is usually accompanied by nausea and sometimes vomiting. Scientists now seem agreed that migraines are connected with changes in blood vessels, in which the vessels first contract and then dilate, causing the pain. Migraines can be one of the side effects of HRT and can be so debilitating that women have to stop taking the hormones.

Food triggers are a major cause of migraine headaches, and this should be the first aspect that is looked at. Foods containing tyramine, nitrite, monosodium glutamate, or alcohol can all be possible suspects. These include chocolate, cheese, and cocoa. Track down whether the migraines are triggered by something you eat or drink by following the recommendations on food allergies in Chapter 10 (see page 181).

Some women get a migraine that is linked to the beginning of their period, and as they reach the menopause these migraines stop. Other women who did not previously have migraines may start to experience them at the onset of the menopause. If you have eliminated any food triggers, it is likely your migraines are hormonal.

As already stated, the liver is the organ of detoxification and gets rid of your ''old'' hormones. If your liver is not functioning properly, these ''old'' hormones can build up like toxins, resulting in a migraine. The same buildup can cause nausea and vomiting without the pain. If you are reacting to certain foods, these will also seem like toxins to your body, so again a migraine and nausea can follow when you eat them.

Nutritional therapy

Eliminate from your diet the major suspect foods that are most likely to be triggering the migraines. See whether you are eating any foods that are overloading your liver, such as coffee, alcohol, or foods high in saturated fat such as cheese. Take:

Quercetin—300mg three times per day
Vitamin C—1000mg twice per day
Vitamin E—300ius per day
Linseed oil capsules—1000mg per day.

SEVEN-DAY LIVER "SPRING-CLEANING"

Because the liver, as our "waste disposal unit," will eliminate toxins and waste products properly when it is working efficiently, we need to keep it functioning in peak condition, especially at the menopause when it is clearing out our "old" hormones. This is a very gentle detox regime. Days 1 to 2: cut out coffee, tea, and alcohol to prepare your body for the cleanse. Days 3 to 7: first thing in the morning, before you have eaten anything, drink this liver "flush" to help your body get rid of toxins and give you a "spring-cleaning." In a blender mix:

1 cup (240 ml.) freshly squeezed lemon juice
1 cup (240 ml.) spring or mineral water
1 clove of fresh garlic
1 tablespoon extra-virgin olive oil
½ in. (1cm.) fresh ginger root.

If you can't drink all that lemon juice, use organic apple juice instead, with a squeeze of lemon. Blend to a smooth liquid and drink slowly.

Drink some apple juice afterward if you have an aftertaste, and fifteen minutes later drink a cup of hot peppermint tea. Then eat normally, but keep your meals very simple so that your body has the chance to eliminate toxins. Eat plenty of fresh fruit and vegetable salads, stir-fried vegetables, vegetable soups, brown rice, oatmeal, etc. You may have headaches or flu-like symptoms for the first couple of days; these are indications that you are detoxifying.

You must eat well to keep your blood sugar up. You can repeat this program every couple of months if you feel you benefit from it.

Herbs

It should be clear from what has gone before (see pages 97–98) that herbal remedies can be very effective in treating the liver, with dandelion and milk thistle at the top of the list. Both these herbs have the ability to help the cleansing process, while milk thistle is also capable of stimulating production of new liver cells.

Feverfew has received a lot of media attention as an "anti-migraine" herb. It really should be used daily as a preventive, rather than taken at the time of an attack. A study at the London Migraine Clinic and reported in the *British Medical Journal* showed remarkable results using this herb.[9]

HEAVY PERIODS (MENORRHAGIA)

You may just naturally have heavy periods. But excessive bleeding could be a symptom of something else that should be investigated. A number of conditions can cause heavy bleeding, including fibroids (benign, harmless growths), endometriosis (the womb lining growing in places other than the womb), pelvic inflammatory disease (an infection), and uterine or cervical cancer. Use of the coil (IUD) for contraception can also be responsible. The cause of the heavy bleeding needs to be checked out first by a doctor.

Fibroids are non-cancerous growths which grow in or on the walls of the uterus of some women and are very common as we get older. It is thought that they actually grow due to an excess of estrogen, so it follows that as we reach the menopause, fibroids may shrink and become less troublesome. They are usually symptomless except for causing heavy periods. They seem to be linked to a later menopause. They can be removed surgically, and often a hysterectomy is advised. Because fibroids are non-cancerous, it makes sense to try natural therapies first to pre-empt the need for what is really major surgery.

The major factor in both heavy bleeding and period pains (see page 109) is the increased production of series 2 prostaglandins. This increase seems to be caused by an increase in arachidonic acid. Arachidonic acid is found predominantly in meat and milk, so by reducing these two foods, along with taking some essential fatty acids (like linseed oil), it is possible to control heavy bleeding and period pains.

Nutritional therapy

If you are bleeding very heavily, you may run the risk of becoming anemic. Take some extra iron, but not in the form of ferrous sulfate. This is an inorganic mineral. Only 2–10 percent of it is actually absorbed by the body, and even then half is eliminated, causing blackening of your stools or constipation. Avoid regular drinking of Indian tea with meals, as this blocks the uptake of iron and other minerals; an herbal tea is perfectly fine.

Vitamin A deficiency has been found in women with heavy periods. By taking good levels of vitamin A, the vast majority of the women in one study in 1977 found the problem eased.[10]

Another study, by Cohen and Rubin, showed that supplementing with vitamin C (200mg three times a day) with bioflavonoids reduced the heavy bleeding in fourteen out of sixteen women.[11] Take:

Vitamin A (as beta-carotene *not* retinol)—10,000ius per day
Zinc citrate or amino acid chelate—15mg per day
Vitamin E—300ius per day
Vitamin C with bioflavonoids—1,000mg, two to three times per day
Iron (as amino acid chelate or citrate)—14mg per day
Vitamin B complex containing 50mg of each B vitamin—once per day

For maximum absorption take the iron with the vitamin C and at a different time from the other supplements.

Herbs

Astringent herbs are usually used because of their ability to regulate blood loss. One such herb, shepherd's purse (*Capsella bursa-pastoris*), has been used in clinical trials to prevent heavy bleeding. Other herbs astringent in nature, and therefore useful for heavy periods, are lady's mantle, yarrow, horsetail, goldenseal, periwinkle, and beth root.

HOT FLASHES/NIGHT SWEATS

These common symptoms are experienced by more than eight out of ten women. You may have a sudden feeling of heat in the face or neck or all over your body. You may wake up with a hot flash at night, bathed in sweat. Women are often very self-conscious about hot flashes, believing that they are obvious to everyone else. They are not usually detectable, but there can be some redness or sweating. One of the major problems with night sweats is that they wake you up, so you feel tired the next day.

Nutritional therapy

This common symptom can be alleviated by taking

Vitamin E—250–400ius per day,
Selenium—15–50mcg. per day,
Vitamin C with bioflavonoids—1–3g. per day.

An interesting study in *Chicago Medicine* showed how much more effective the bioflavonoids and vitamin C were for controlling hot flashes compared with HRT.[12] The researchers looked at thirty-six women who had gone into menopause as a result of surgery and fifty-eight whose menopause had come naturally. The vitamin C and bioflavonoids had a dramatic and positive effect in stopping or reducing the hot flashes. The researchers also put forward an interesting theory as to why this happened. Normally circulating estrogen keeps our blood vessels toned and prevents excessive vasodilation (opening of the blood vessels which makes us sweat). The suggestion is that the vitamin C and bioflavonoids that are taken as our estrogen levels drop help tonify the blood vessels and so lessen the hot flashes.

A number of studies have shown the benefits of vitamin E supplementation in helping to control hot flashes.[13] In one study, a group of women who had been taking the vitamin E supplement, and whose hot flashes had gone, were then switched to a placebo (dummy pill) without their knowledge. The hot flashes returned.

Herbs

Vitex is by far the most potent remedy for hot flashes and night sweats as it contains the chemical building blocks of the sex hormones. It does not contain any actual hormones, so it is safe to use without the risk of causing an imbalance. It is very effective for relieving hot flashes. Black cohosh, a herb used by Native Americans, is very effective in restoring female hormonal balance and helps relieve menopausal symptoms. Other herbs, such as dong quai, licorice, and alfalfa have all been shown to have beneficial estrogenic effect. Yarrow, which is known as a prime fever remedy because of its ability to lower body temperature, is ideal for taking during the hot flashes and night sweats of the menopause.

Aromatherapy

Dilute 15 drops of Roman chamomile into 1fl. oz. (25ml.) of carrier oil composed of two parts sweet almond oil and one part wheatgerm oil.

Roman chamomile (not German chamomile) is an adaptogen, so it helps the body balance itself. Use the oil for a wonderful massage, or simply sniff during the day if you start to feel symptoms developing.

LOW LIBIDO

Lack of interest in sex may have a great deal to do with just feeling tired. Follow the recommendations for lack of energy to see if that makes a difference. If we are tired, the only thing we can think about when we get to bed is going to sleep!

Lower estrogen levels, of course, are often blamed for lack of interest in sex. But is this true? It's interesting to note that while most women are told about falling levels of estrogen and progesterone, nobody ever mentions testosterone. This is the "male" hormone linked with male characteristics such as a deep voice and greater body hair, and is also connected to drive and motivation. But women have testosterone circulating in their bodies too, and it has been found that as we enter the menopause the level of this hormone can drop. However, some women actually register an increase in testosterone at this time, and these women feel their sex drive has actually increased, not fallen at all.

Nutritional therapy

Take:

  Magnesium—300mg per day
  Zinc—15–30mg per day
  Vitamin B6—take as 50mg pyridoxal-5-phosphate once
    per day.

Herbs

American ginseng is effective in increasing energy levels. Other herbs that normalize hormone balance can be used, such as vitex and black cohosh.

Aromatherapy

Add 7 drops of damiana and 7 drops of geranium to a carrier oil. Damiana is a well-known herbal aphrodisiac.

MEMORY/CONCENTRATION

Poor memory, lack of concentration, impaired hearing, and ringing in the ears are often caused by an obstructed blood supply to the brain. But this may be a problem to do with age rather than hormones. Our brain's "food" is the oxygen supplied by the blood. Logically, we can see that if the blood supply is deficient, our mental function can be impaired. Brain cells alone account for 25 percent of the body's total oxygen consumption. As we age, we can also experience dizzy spells, as well as cold hands and feet, often a result of poor blood circulation.

With memory, as with the sexual side of our lives, it can be a case of "use it or lose it." It is important that you keep mentally active. Our brains have been likened to a container or pot which we can never fill up. It is similar to our muscles. If we were bedridden for a number of months without using our muscles, we would find it very difficult to walk when we finally got up and tried. It has been suggested that we use only about 10 percent of our brain capacity. The more we use our brains, the more interconnections we make, and the easier it is to remember and concentrate.

Nutritional therapy

Hardening of the arteries can be the cause of this reduced blood supply to the brain, so it is important that we keep the saturated fat content of our diet low. This hardening (arteriosclerosis) is caused by an accumulation of fats and the buildup of cholesterol in the arteries which causes them to narrow and so restrict blood flow. The process is similar to the furring-up of a pipe, with the opening becoming smaller and smaller as the deposits increase. Eat well, as for the menopause generally, and include plenty of fresh fruit and vegetables in your diet. Take:

Vitamin C—1,000mg twice per day
Vitamin B6—50mg per day

Vitamin E—300ius once per day
Magnesium—300mg per day
Selenium—25mcg per day

Herbs

Ginkgo biloba tree leaf extract is now believed to have a rejuvenating effect on the brain. Several clinical trials have shown that it helps improve learning ability, concentration, and memory. An article in *The Lancet* concluded that ginkgo biloba

- improves blood flow to the head
- increases the supply of glucose and oxygen which the brain needs to create energy
- prevents blood clots
- protects the brain cells against damage

PAINFUL PERIODS (DYSMENORRHEA)

First make sure there is no other underlying cause for the pain (e.g. endometriosis, infection, etc.). Endometriosis is a condition in which the lining of the womb (the endometrium) grows in places other than the womb itself. These tissues bleed during periods and can cause severe pain. When you have checked that there is no organic cause for the pain, you may find that natural remedies make a real difference to painful periods.

Nutritional therapy

Both magnesium and calcium work as muscle relaxants, so it is worth supplementing with them. Take a good multi-vitamin and mineral supplement with a reasonable amount of calcium, then add the extra amounts below and see if that is sufficient. If you are still having pain after a few weeks, you may need to add in extra calcium through a combined magnesium and calcium supplement. Reduce your intake of animal foods to keep the arachidonic acid production under control. Take:

Magnesium—300mg. per day
Linseed oil capsules—100mg. per day
Vitamin E—300ius per day
Vitamin C with bioflavonoids—1,000mg. twice per day
Zinc citrate—15mg. per day.

Herbs

Some herbs can help to relax muscles and stop abdominal cramps. Others can help to balance the female hormones.

Cramp bark, with its wonderful name, really works as an antispasmodic and muscle relaxant. Another herb which is very similar to cramp bark and also useful for period pains is blackhaw.

Besides taking away the pain, it is wise to address the cause of the period pains by combining one of the muscle relaxants with a good hormone balancer. As in the case of hot flashes, vitex is a good normalizer for the hormones. It is safe to use because it helps regulate the hormones without introducing an external hormone.

A good mixture for painful periods is equal parts of skullcap, blackhaw, and black cohosh taken at a dosage of 5ml (1 teaspoon) three times a day when needed.

SKIN PROBLEMS

Skin problems such as dry skin, eczema, psoriasis, acne, itching, and skin rashes can often be due to a poorly functioning liver, and you may need professional help from a nutritional therapist to deal with this. Food allergies have also been linked with skin problems, so it would be worth looking at your diet to see if anything you eat or drink could be responsible. A way for you to do this yourself is explained in Chapter 10 (see page 181).

Nutritional therapy

Reduce your intake of saturated fats, and eat a good, varied diet. Include plenty of foods that contain essential fatty acids, such as oily fish, nuts, seeds, and oils.
Take:

Zinc—up to 30mg. per day
Vitamin B complex containing 100mg. of each B vitamin—once per day
Linseed oil capsules—up to 1,000mg. per day.

Herbs

Burdock root has been used successfully for skin problems for many years, especially for eczema. It is useful for dry and scaly skin and is also effective for dandruff. Other herbs that are good for the skin are echinacea, cleavers, red clover, and nettle. Studies have shown that herbs (such as licorice and German chamomile) applied directly to the skin can be just as effective as, or even more effective than, the cortiscone drug treatment that doctors sometimes recommend. Topical herbs (i.e. herbs applied to the skin) are useful to give temporary relief, but the underlying causes of the skin problem should always be addressed internally.

SLEEP PROBLEMS

Sleep problems can be quite different from insomnia. I see many women who have no difficulty in getting to sleep but then find themselves waking in the night. This can happen just once in the very early hours of the morning or a number of times during the course of the night. And it may be a struggle to get back to sleep again.

This can be a common symptom at the menopause due to night sweats. If you are waking during the night because you are sweating, then your sleep will be disturbed and you will feel tired the next morning. It is important to use the recommendations for controlling hot flashes/night sweats first. If those do not work, you may have a more general sleep problem.

Insomnia should be tackled physically and mentally. Sometimes we are not sleeping because our minds are so active that our thoughts just go round and round. It is important to look at the dietary side too, since that is the easiest to control. Your sleep problems may be solved by adjusting what you eat and drink. If not, then it is time to take control of your mind.

Before going to bed you can have a relaxing warm bath with essential oils such as bergamot, lavender, or chamomile. There are a number of good relaxing bath oils already made up and ready to use which are easily available in stores. Learn a relaxation technique which you can practice in bed, such as tensing and relaxing each part of your body in turn. Or try a visualization technique. Imagine yourself on a beautiful beach with the warm sun on your skin, soft sand under your feet, blue sky, clear water, and the fragrant scent all around you from wonderful colored flowers. In the distance you can hear the sounds of birds, and there is a gentle breeze in the palm trees. You have nothing to do and no cares in the world—just let yourself go. You can tape this visualization for yourself to play while you go to sleep, or you can buy a prerecorded relaxation tape.

Because our mental and physical states are so intertwined, they feed off each other, positively and negatively. If something is worrying us, our bodies become tense and unable to relax. This makes sleep more difficult, which in turn makes us even more stressed. If something physical is stopping us from sleeping, we feel worried and agitated and then our bodies become even more tense and tight.

BLACKBOARD TECHNIQUE

This is a good way of getting to sleep. It's a variation on counting sheep—but much more effective.

❑ Lying in bed with your eyes closed, imagine a blackboard. Picture yourself with a piece of chalk in one hand and an eraser in the other.

❑ Draw a large circle. Inside the circle put the number 100.

❑ Use the eraser to rub out the number, but be careful not to rub out the circle. When you have finished, write the number 99, rub it out as before and continue indefinitely.

❑ Even if you realize that you've gone back to thinking again, just stop and start from the last number you can remember.

The mind becomes bored with this routine and eventually shuts down. As you do this exercise each night you should find yourself going to sleep more and more quickly because the mind becomes bored with the routine sooner. It can get to the point that you only have to think about the blackboard and the mind tells you, "Oh no, not again, sleep is preferable to this," and shuts down. If you wake in the night, use the blackboard technique, or go to the bathroom, and then come back to bed and use the technique.

Nutritional therapy

First, have a close look at what you are eating and drinking during the day. Cut out all the stimulants such as coffee, tea, sugar, chocolate, etc., and make sure you eat little and often without going over three hours without food. Some women find themselves waking up at 3 to 4 a.m., sometimes quite abruptly and with palpitations. This is caused by the blood sugar level dropping overnight. As the blood sugar level gets low, the body is releasing adrenaline into the bloodstream to try to correct this imbalance. So at 3 to 4 in the morning there is a huge surge of adrenaline and you wake up with no idea what's caused it.

Have a cup of chamomile tea before going to bed to help with sleep problems.

Magnesium is known as "nature's tranquilizer," so it's a good mineral supplement for helping with sleep problems. You could take one dose about an hour before going to bed. If you take B vitamins, try to take them in the early part of the day, not after lunch. A number of women whom I have seen who have taken B vitamins to increase their energy levels found they couldn't go to sleep when they took them in the afternoon or evening. If you suffer from restless legs in bed, both magnesium and vitamin E can be very helpful. Take:

Magnesium—250mg. per day
Vitamin E—300ius per day.

Herbs

Herbs really come into their own here, because they are so effective at helping us to relax naturally.

Valerian has been used for centuries to assist with sleep problems, and its powers to prevent insomnia and improve sleep quality have been confirmed in studies. Ordinary sleeping pills can leave you feeling hungover and sleepy in the morning, but valerian doesn't usually have this inconvenient side effect at all. It is classed as a sedative in herbal medicine and can be used to reduce tension and anxiety and promote natural sleep.

Passionflower or passiflora is another good herb for helping you sleep. It is thought that this herb contains alkaloids which work directly on the central nervous system to ensure restful sleep. It can be combined with valerian to give a very effective remedy for sleep problems without an addictive effect.

STRESS INCONTINENCE

Stress incontinence is the leaking of a small amount of urine when you laugh, cough, or sneeze. It can be embarrassing and inconvenient, and women often don't want to tell even their doctors about it. It is thought to be linked to the menopause because estrogen helps to keep the sphincter muscle at the base of the bladder tight. As estrogen declines, the muscle can become weak.

Kegel exercises can strengthen the pelvic muscles, including those of the vagina. These exercises can be done at any time because nobody knows you are doing them. All you do is draw the vaginal muscles firmly inward and upward, hold for a count of five, and then relax. These are the same muscles that you would use to stop the flow of urine in midstream, when you have to give a sample. You may remember being urged to do these pelvic floor exercises when you were expecting a baby. They should be a part of every woman's exercise program, whatever her age. If stress incontinence becomes a real problem, and you have tried a number of complementary practices including acupuncture to no avail, there are cones available on the market which can be inserted in the vagina to help strengthen the muscles.

Nutritional therapy

Eat well and follow the recommendations in the chapter on nutrition (see page 42), so that you are making the most of your own circulating estrogen to keep the muscles taut.

Vitamin C is important in stress incontinence because its major function is to produce collagen. Collagen is the most abundant protein in the body and gives strength to tissues. Take:

Vitamin C—1,000mg. three times per day.

Herbs

Herbs for stress incontinence focus on strengthening the kidneys and include dandelion root, rehmannia, chickweed, marshmallow, ginkgo, astralagus, and urva ursi (also known as bearberry).

VAGINAL DRYNESS

As hormone levels change at the menopause, the vagina is affected. There is a tendency for the vaginal walls to become narrower and thinner and for the level of natural secretions accompanying sexual arousal to fall, which can make intercourse uncomfortable. This is another one of those "use it or lose it" situations. During lovemaking and orgasm, blood circulation is increased in the vagina, and this can revive the vaginal tissues. It is important to keep up a good intake of essential fatty acids in your food and not to go on a "no fat" diet, as you need the lubrication from these oils.

A study in a gynecological journal showed that supplementing with vitamin E produced positive changes in the blood vessels in the vaginal walls after only four weeks.[14] I have found insertion of vitamin E to be more successful than taking it orally, hence the recommendation below.

Nutritional therapy

Insert a vitamin E capsule inside your vagina every night for six weeks, and after this time just use as you feel you need it.

Herbs

Herbs such as vitex which help to normalize the hormones at the menopause will be useful here. Motherwort can help by restoring thickness and elasticity to the vaginal walls. The Chinese herb dong quai is also useful for vaginal dryness. If the dryness is affecting your relationship with your partner or making sex very uncomfortable, it may be better to seek professional help from a herbalist or a practitioner with a good working knowledge of herbs to obtain more detailed advice on how to cope with the hormone changes affecting your vagina.

WATER RETENTION

This is a common symptom for many women who suffer swelling and bloating, and often it is worst just before a period. It can be so bad you may have trouble getting rings on fingers, and your shoes on your feet.

Nutritional therapy

Your first instinct may be to limit the amount you drink. This is a mistake. In fact it's the opposite of what you actually need to do. You should drink more water and reduce your intake of salt and of hidden salt in convenience foods. If you limit your intake of water, your body will think there is a shortage of water and try to retain what you have, hence the swelling.

Many women who suffer from water retention turn to diuretics. Diuretics will increase the rate at which you lose fluids, but you will also lose important minerals which will be flushed out of your body at the same time. Potassium is one of the minerals that you may lose, but it is vital in the correct functioning of your heart. Take:

Vitamin C—1,000mg twice per day
Linseed capsules—1,000mg twice per day
Vitamin B6—50mg per day
Vitamin E—300ius per day
Magnesium—150mg per day.

Herbs

An interesting experiment with animals looked at the effect on body weight produced by taking the herb dandelion. The animals lost 30 percent of their original weight when given the herb. The researchers felt this was due to the release of water retention.[15]

Dandelion is a natural diuretic which allows fluid to be released without losing vital nutrients at the same time. Dandelion itself contains more vitamins and minerals than any other herb and is one of the best natural sources of potassium.

Parsley, rich in vitamin C, is also useful as a diuretic. If the aim is to help reduce water retention, taking it in tincture form gives the most effective results. It is important also to make sure that your hormones are in balance and to use it in conjunction with normalizing herbs such as vitex and black cohosh.

Aromatherapy

Fennel is very effective in countering water retention. Add 10 drops to a warm bath and soak in it for fifteen to twenty minutes. Then massage your body using 15 drops of fennel.

Main herbs for the menopause

Vitex (*agnus castus*, chasteberry) This is a popular herb at the menopause because it stimulates and normalizes the function of the pituitary gland, which controls and balances the hormones in our body. So vitex works to restore balance and is used where there is a hormone deffcit as well as where there is a hormone excess. Uses:

- regulates periods,
- helps with heavy bleeding or too-frequent periods,
- alleviates premenstrual symptoms,
- helps with painful periods,
- reduces hot flashes,
- can increase the ratio of progesterone to estrogen by balancing excess estrogen.

Black cohosh (*Cimicifuga racemosa*) This herb has long been used by Native Americans. Like vitex it is another good normalizer for the female hormone system. Uses:

- helps with painful periods,
- helps regain hormone balance,
- reduces hot flashes,
- helps with premenstrual symptoms,
- reduces water retention.

Blue cohosh (*Caulophyllum thalictroides*) This herb, too, is used by Native Americans and is sometimes called squaw or papoose root. Uses:

- helps regulate periods,
- helps where there is a weakness or loss of tone in the womb.

False unicorn root (*Chamaelirium luteum*) Another North American herb—a good tonic and strengthener for the reproductive system. Use:

- has a balancing effect on the hormones.

Yarrow (*Achillea millefolium*) This herb is known as the ideal fever remedy because it has the ability to lower the body temperature. Uses:

- alleviates hot flashes and night sweats,
- alleviates heavy bleeding,
- helps with painful periods.

Dandelion (*Taraxacum officinale*) This herb helps to cleanse the liver—the organ of detoxification which also helps to get rid of accumulated "old" female hormones. If the liver is functioning effectively, this prevents excess estrogen from building up, so reducing the risk of breast growths and other cell changes. Use:

- reduces water retention.

Motherwort (*Leonurus cardiaca*) This is a very good herb for the reproductive system. Uses:

- alleviates painful periods,
- reduces hot flashes,
- helps to calm anxiety at the menopause,
- helps combat insomnia,
- alleviates vaginal dryness—restoring thickness and elasticity to the vaginal walls.

Dong quai (*Radix angelica sinensis*) This Oriental herb is the one most frequently used for menstrual complaints. It is extensively cultivated in Asia for medicinal purposes and in traditional Chinese medicine is well-known as a tonic for the female reproductive system. Uses:

• alleviates period pains,
• regulates periods,
• reduces spotting,
• reduces hot flashes/night sweats,
• alleviates vaginal dryness.

Wild Yam (*Dioscorea villosa*) The role of this herb needs to be explained because the media seem to have confused it with progesterone. Estrogen and progesterone have been synthesized from wild yam—at one time this was the only source of raw material for the contraceptive pill. But wild yam, the plant, does not contain these hormones at all. Traditional herbalists would not choose wild yam to alleviate menopausal symptoms. It has always been valued for its antispasmodic qualities, which make it helpful in the treatment of painful periods and muscle pains and as an anti-inflammatory in the treatment of rheumatoid arthritis.

Our bodies cannot produce progesterone from wild yam: that can be done only in a laboratory. But it seems that the disogenin in the herb is able to copy the effects of estrogen in our bodies. When blood estrogen levels are high, wild yam is theoretically able to reduce estrogen activity, and conversely, when estrogen levels are low, it is able to promote estrogen activity. In other words the herb works as a balancer and will do only what is appropriate at the time. This is quite different from taking progesterone or estrogen derived from wild yam (or from any outside source), which results in the body's supply of one hormone being boosted whether it needs it or not.

Conclusion

There are many good readymade herbal mixtures available which are designed for the menopause. They contain a number of the herbs mentioned above which have been found to be most effective for menopausal symptoms. You will get the greatest benefit by choosing a combination of remedies, because certain herbs will work better for some women than others. By taking a variety of herbs and getting a mixture, you are actually covering all possibilities and increasing the potential efficacy of the remedy.

CHAPTER 7

What is osteoporosis?

Most women are aware of osteoporosis as a potentially debilitating bone condition which can lead to fractures of the wrist, spine, and hip in later years. You may have read or been told that Hormone Replacement Therapy is recommended as a prime protection against thinning bones. But the fact is that a good diet, along with nutritional supplements and exercise, is the best way of preventing osteoporosis. Osteoporosis literally means porous bones—bones that are filled with tiny holes. Our bones are not static. Formed primarily from calcium, they are in a constant state of change. Bone is continuously broken down and rebuilt through the body's biochemical processes. Two kinds of cells are important for this process, osteoclasts and osteoblasts. Osteoclasts renew old bone by dissolving or resorbing it, leaving an empty space. The osteoblasts then fill this empty space with new bone.

Bone loss results when the rate of renewal does not equal the rate of breakdown, and this can result in osteoporosis. The dense outer bone is called the cortical layer, while underneath this is the trabecular or spongy layer. Cortical bone is renewed completely every ten to twelve years. Trabecular bone has a much faster turnover, and there is complete renewal every two to three years. Our wrists, thighs, and vertebrae contain mostly trabecular bone, and the most common fractures occur in these parts, although the vertebrae are more protected because of their shape, which adds strength.

Bones don't actually change shape with osteoporosis. The loss is within the bone, making it spongy and more likely to break. Often the first sign of osteoporosis is a fracture following a relatively minor stress or accident. It has even been suggested that the bone breaks first and then the fall happens because of the weakness caused by the break. The fact that osteoporosis may not be diagnosed until after a fracture is a frightening prospect for women. In fact the bone mass of both men and women naturally decreases as they get older. It starts declining in our mid thirties, and the rate of decline increases during the ten years around the time of the menopause before slowing down again.

Osteoporosis and the menopause

The popular theory is that women are at risk of developing brittle bones at the menopause because of lower estrogen levels. Estrogen, it is true, helps stimulate the liver to produce a protein that protects the bones against the harmful dissolving effects of adrenaline. But it's clear that this is not the whole picture. If the estrogen theory is correct, why do men, who have relatively small amounts of estrogen in their bodies all their lives, not suffer more from osteoporosis than women? Men tend to have only a fraction of the bone density loss experienced by women. In tests it has been found that the male hormone testosterone triggers the bone-building osteoblasts, and this is accompanied by higher levels of the enzyme alkaline phosphatase, which helps to form calcium crystals in the bone. As we reach the menopause, and our ovaries reduce their production of estrogen, we then have proportionately more testosterone circulating in our system. It is possible that if we are in optimum health, our bodies provide fail-safe mechanisms to take over as one set of hormones reduces.

And bone density loss in women is not universal. Research has demonstrated that Asian and Caucasian women are more likely to suffer bone loss than African women, for instance. In Singapore more men than women get osteoporosis, while in Hong Kong they seem to be equally susceptible. And why does bone mass start to decline when we are in our thirties, when estrogen levels should still be high? Research demonstrates that bone loss starts well *before* the menopause and *before* any decreases in estrogen levels. The anti-estrogen drug Tamoxifen is given to women at risk of breast cancer. If lack of estrogen is the prime cause of osteoporosis, it would be logical to expect that Tamoxifen would cause bone loss. But this does not seem to be a side effect.[1]

A few years ago there was a fascinating article in the British medical journal *The Lancet* about tests done on eighteenth-century human bones discovered during the restoration of a London church.[2] The rate of bone loss in modern women, both pre- and post-menopause was found to be far higher than that apparently experienced by our ancestors. All this suggests that estrogen levels are not the only, nor the most important, factor in bone loss. It seems to indicate that differences in lifestyles, what we eat—or what we don't eat—are a crucial element in the complex process of bone manufacture. This means that serious bone loss is not an inevitable part of the menopause, although the menopause may accelerate it. It is something that we ourselves can take positive action about without resorting to very powerful hormone drugs through fear. But first we need to understand a little more about what is going on.

The calcium factor

"Drink up your milk." Probably the first health "fact" we are ever told is that calcium-rich foods are good for our bones and teeth. Nowadays the message is that calcium-rich foods, or calcium supplements, will help prevent osteoporosis. Well, up to a point. Ninety-nine percent of the body's calcium is certainly stored in our bones. Bone is a living, hard, yet flexible tissue made up of small crystals of calcium, phosphorus, and other minerals held together by collagen. The crystals give our bones strength. The bones need constant supplies of calcium for renewal. But there is more to it than that. What puts calcium into bones and what takes it out? We may be taking in sufficient calcium but not enough is necessarily being deposited in our bones. Too much may be excreted in our urine. We must indeed replenish our calcium supplies—but we must also make sure we are not depleting our stores of calcium unnecessarily at the same time. It's one thing putting calcium-rich food in our mouths; getting it into our bones is a different matter, and one that is all too frequently glossed over by snappy headlines and the glib advice dished out to women. There is a lot more involved in the process.

When we eat food containing calcium, we need both stomach acid (hydrochloric acid) and vitamin D in order to absorb that calcium properly. The calcium is incorporated in our bones by the action of a hormone, calcitonin. If our blood levels of calcium drop, another substance, parathyroid hormone, reabsorbs calcium from our bones and circulates it in the blood to right the imbalance. So this process is dependent on two opposite-acting hormones, calcitonin and parathyroid hormone, which keep our blood calcium in balance. If there is insufficient calcitonin, not enough calcium can be deposited in our bones. If there is excess parathyroid hormone, too much calcium can be taken out. Estrogen stops the latter hormone going about its business of taking calcium from bone to rebalance the amount in the blood. This is one reason why women are constantly told that the estrogen in HRT provides protection against osteoporosis. In a narrow sense this is true. But it does not address the fundamental issue of maintaining the all-important calcium balance.

The key to healthy bones lies in maintaining this delicate calcium balance, and here our diet is absolutely crucial.

The acid factor

Calcium's role in the body is to act as a neutralizer. When we eat too much acid food, our own reserves of calcium from bones and teeth are called up to correct the imbalance. The term "acid foods" probably brings to mind things like grapefruit and oranges. But "acidic" in this context describes the effect of food on the body and the calcium balance. It is what the food becomes once you have eaten it

---

Functions of the bone hormones

Calcitonin

Production is stimulated by high calcium and magnesium in the blood. It

- acts on osteoblasts (builds new bones),
- decreases blood calcium levels,
- stops release of calcium from the bones.

Parathyroid

Production is stimulated by low calcium and magnesium in the blood. It

- acts on osteoclasts (dissolves old bone),
- increases blood calcium levels,
- triggers the release of calcium from the bones.

Estrogen stops its production.

---

that is important. When you have finished digesting and absorbing a food, there is a residue left called ash, and it is the quality of this ash that determines whether a food is acid or alkali. Fruits, including citrus fruits and vegetables, are alkaline-forming whereas foods containing animal protein, such as milk, cheese, meat, chicken, and fish, are acid-forming.

So if you are continually eating a diet that is too acid, you will continually be using up your stores of calcium. It doesn't matter how much calcium you are taking in through food or supplements, if you are leeching the body of its calcium stores, you are facing a losing battle. So you must *stop* using up so much calcium in the first place. The main foods that cause an acid reaction are proteins—animal proteins in particular. It has been estimated that for every extra ⅓ oz. (10g.) of protein we eat, 100mg. of calcium is lost in our urine. Western diets are very dependent on animal protein and are therefore acidic.

It makes sense, therefore, to omit meat from some of your meals. Or make more use of vegetable proteins such as tofu or nuts. A 147-pound (67kg.) person needs no more than 1½ oz. (40g.) of protein a day. The link between protein and calcium loss has been known to scientists for over fifty years. But even today, when someone announces that he or she is going to become vegetarian they are greeted with shrill cries of "But where are you going to get your protein from?" One study of 1,600 women showed that the vegetarians had only 18 percent bone mass loss compared to the 35 percent experienced by meat eaters. In the animal kingdom some of the large, strong-boned mammals like giraffes and elephants are grass eaters.[3]

Excess calcium

We all hear a lot from the media about the need to take more calcium. It's never pointed out that too much of a good thing can be bad for you. You can have too much calcium. Too much calcium can lead to painful kidney stones, loss of appetite, and abdominal pains. Too much calcium continually circulating in the blood means that it may be deposited in places other than in the bone. Calcification of soft tissue, for instance, can cause arteriosclerosis (thickness of the arteries). In nature balance is all. Too much or too little of anything can damage your overall health. Because it is virtually impossible for us to control that balance on a daily basis and to know we are getting it right, we need to give our bodies the chance to balance themselves. By giving ourselves optimum health through natural measures and a proper diet, we are giving ourselves that opportunity.

Are you at risk from osteoporosis?

According to some estimates, as many as one in three women will suffer from osteoporosis. It's difficult to know quite what that means. Most women (and men) will suffer some bone mass loss as they age. But in reality it's hard to predict who will be so severely affected that they suffer fractures. Osteoporosis is said to have reached "epidemic" proportions. But how many people do you actually know who suffer from it? Many people suffer bone mass loss without its being a problem. There are, however, some known factors that seem to indicate higher-than-average risk of severe bone mass loss and fractures in later life. These factors are heredity, premature menopause, inactivity, smoking, alcohol and coffee, drugs and medicines, irregular periods, weight, and faulty digestion.

HEREDITY

Heredity is now believed to be a major factor in osteoporosis. Advances in research have shown that a number of inherited genes may put some women at greater risk. The latest scientific breakthrough has come from comparing sets of non-identical with identical twins. Identical twins have exactly the same genes—non-identical twins do not. So it's possible to isolate genetic factors from environmental and other differences when comparing medical histories. Research is in the early stages, but it is suspected that one defective gene may prevent the body from using vitamin D efficiently, while another may prevent the absorption of estrogen. Many experts have believed for some time that a woman whose mother (or father) has osteoporosis may be at higher risk herself. But although you were born with an inherited constitution, your own lifestyle and diet can weaken or strengthen your inherited health characteristics.

PREMATURE MENOPAUSE

A premature menopause is one that occurs before the age of forty, but it can happen to women in their twenties. There may be no definite cause, but it can be due to radiotherapy given to treat cancer or to surgical removal of the ovaries because of disease. In a premature or surgical menopause the estrogen levels fall off sharply instead of undergoing the gradual decline you normally expect at menopause. The sudden low levels of estrogen may be linked to a greater risk of osteoporosis.

INACTIVITY

It's well known that astronauts lose some of their bone density while they are in space. The theory is that in a gravity-free environment the body does not need to support itself, so it stops increasing bone density. Therefore again the motto is: "Use it or lose it." This may be another reason why osteoporosis could be considered a modern life-style complaint. Just as weightlessness appears to cause bone loss, making few demands on our joints and limbs robs our bones of the ability to build up and maintain strength. In a sedentary society we need to make the effort to get enough of the right exercise. Weight-bearing exercises increase bone density in the lower limbs and arms. Just taking moderate exercise has been shown to increase bone density in post-menopausal women.[4] Maintaining physical fitness also tones up the muscles and improves the protective responses of the muscles around the hips. Hip fracture is the most common fracture in women. Strengthening your muscles makes you better able to absorb the force of a fall. Being physically fit improves coordination and flexibility, making you less likely to fall in the first place. Research at Nottingham University, in England, has shown that doing just fifty jumps a day makes hip bones more dense.

SMOKING

Smoking seems to change the pattern of the female hormones into one more normally seen at the menopause, with lower levels of estrogen. Low levels of estrogen are thought to be linked to osteoporosis, so smokers are not only at higher risk but are also likely to get the condition earlier than non-smokers. It has been shown that smoking can reduce bone mass by up to 25 percent.

ALCOHOL AND COFFEE

There are several reasons why a high intake of alcohol or coffee increases the risk of osteoporosis. Both cause extreme changes in blood sugar levels (for a more detailed explanation see Chapter 5). Essentially the drop in blood sugar causes the release of adrenaline in the body to help restore the balance by using our own sugar stores. Excess adrenaline has been shown to dissolve bone. Estrogen can help prevent this, but at the menopause we do not have the same amounts of estrogen which would have previously protected us.

Coffee causes an acid reaction. So calcium in its role as neutralizer will be taken from your bones in order to balance that acid (see page 125). You deplete your own supplies of calcium and risk your bone health. A recent American study showed that drinking more than two cups of coffee or four cups of tea a day increased the risk of hip fractures.[5] Another study showed that people who drank more than three cups of coffee each day increased their risk of osteoporosis by 82 percent.

A high intake of alcohol weakens your liver, a major organ of detoxification which gets rid of toxins and also waste hormones. It also produces a protein that protects your bone against the harmful dissolving effects of adrenaline. If your liver is compromised, it will not be able to produce this protein effectively, and so the adrenaline is free to attack your bones.

DRUGS AND MEDICINES

Certain drugs are known to accelerate the rate of bone mass loss. Women who need to take corticosteroids because of a chronic inflammatory disorder should be monitored carefully since there is a risk of bone mass loss when taking this medication. But frequent use of laxatives and diuretics can also put you at risk because calcium and other essential nutrients are flushed out of the body. If you are taking thyroxin because of an underactive thyroid, you have a greater risk of developing osteoporosis. You should have your bone density checked and also make sure that you are not being given more thyroxin than you actually need.[6] More thyroxin than you actually require may result in a seven times greater loss of bone density.

IRREGULAR PERIODS

This means that your hormones are not circulating in the body as they should. In one study women with a history of irregular menstruation before the age of forty had an average loss in bone density of more than 8 percent compared to women with regular periods.[7]

WEIGHT

Women never actually stop producing estrogen in their bodies. At the menopause, when our ovaries slow down, the production of estrogen from our fat cells takes over and manufactures a form of the hormone to supplement this loss. Not surprisingly it is now believed that being the right weight for your height is very important in ensuring that you have enough fat for the production of this estrogen. The body mass index (BMI), a ratio of height to weight, is the best way to determine this.

To calculate your BMI, use the charts opposite to calculate your height in meters and your weight in kilograms:

BMI = your weight in kg. divided by the square of your height in meters. For example, if my weight is 140 pounds (63.5kg.) and my height is 5ft. 6in. (1.68m.), my BMI =

$$\frac{63.5}{1.68 \times 1.68} = 22.5$$

A number of studies have shown that the BMI is a reliable indicator of osteoporosis risk.[8] One indicated that when the BMI fell from twenty-five to twenty there was a seven-fold increase in risk.[9] Another demonstrated that women aged forty-five to fifty-nine who had suffered fractures had an average BMI of 22.5, while those without fractures had an average BMI of 25.3.[10] The BMI was still a

Weight					
Lb.	Kg.	Lb.	Kg.	Lb.	Kg.
110	50	134	60.8	158	71.7
111	50.5	135	61.2	159	72.2
112	50.8	136	61.7	160	72.6
113	51.3	137	62.1	161	73.1
114	51.7	138	62.6	162	73.5
115	52.2	139	63.1	163	74.0
116	52.6	140	63.5	164	74.4
117	53.1	141	64.0	165	74.9
118	53.5	142	64.4	166	75.3
119	54.0	143	64.9	167	75.8
120	54.4	144	65.3	168	76.2
121	54.9	145	65.8	169	76.7
122	55.3	146	66.2	170	77.1
123	55.8	147	66.7	171	77.6
124	56.3	148	67.1	172	78.0
125	56.7	149	67.6	173	78.5
126	57.2	150	68.0	174	78.9
127	57.6	151	68.5	175	79.4
128	58.1	152	69.0	176	79.8
129	58.5	153	69.4	177	80.3
130	59.0	154	69.9	178	80.7
131	59.4	155	70.4	179	81.2
132	59.9	156	70.8	180	81.6
133	60.3	157	71.3		

Height					
ft. in.	m.	ft. in.	m.	ft. in.	m.
4 10	1.47	5 3	1.60	5 8	1.73
4 11	1.50	5 4	1.63	5 9	1.75
5 0	1.52	5 5	1.65	5 10	1.78
5 1	1.55	5 6	1.68	5 11	1.80
5 2	1.57	5 7	1.70	6 0	1.83

good indicator as the women got older. Those aged sixty-five to seventy-five with hip fractures had a BMI of 21 while healthy women of the same age had an average BMI of 24.6. As the BMI falls, bone density declines even in the absence of fractures. Losing a significant amount of weight quickly may be particularly relevant to loss of bone mass.

FAULTY DIGESTION

As we get older we produce less stomach acid (hydrochloric acid), and this can interfere with the proper absorption of calcium and other nutrients from our food. Hydrochloric acid helps the absorption of dietary calcium, and vitamin D is necessary to incorporate calcium into bone. If food passes through your system too rapidly, as may be the case if you suffer from irritable bowel syndrome, this can also upset calcium absorption.

Tests for bone density

Anyone who believes they are at risk from osteoporosis can find out what is happening to their bones. There are tests available that enable you to monitor bone loss over the years. Ask your doctor about this.

DUAL ENERGY X-RAY ABSORPTIOMETRY

This is the most widely used technique for measuring bone mineral density. It is a scanner which uses two simultaneous X-ray energy beams, one high energy and the other low energy. The low-energy beam can pass through soft tissue but not bone. Bone density can be calculated from how much energy the bone and soft tissues absorb from the energy beam. The scanner can measure bone mineral density at multiple points on your body. This is important, since bone mineral density at one site does not necessarily reflect the situation at other points. With osteoporosis the earliest bone loss typically starts in the trabecular bones, such as the spine and hip, so these are important sites to test if you think you are at risk. The disadvantage of this test is that you are exposing yourself to X-rays, and this can be cumulative if you want to monitor your bones over the years. It has a 1 percent error rate.

PHOTON ABSORPTIOMETRY

An alternative to X-rays is the use of a very high-intensity light. Two or more measures over time are required to determine bone loss rates. The disadvantage is that the test cannot be used on the spine. This technique has an 8 percent error rate.

ULTRASOUND

High-speed sound waves pass painlessly through the heel-bone, giving vital information about bone density structure and risk of fracture within two minutes. But only the heel is measured, and it is assumed that this is representative of your bone in general, which may not be the case. No X-rays are involved, so repeated monitoring carries no risk.

URINE ANALYSIS

This is a simple non-invasive test which measures bone resorption. It can identify current levels of bone loss and the risk of future loss. Because it measures the biochemical processes of bone formation, it is a good way of monitoring the effects of diet and nutritional supplements. The test measures the presence of pyridinium and deoxypyridinium—two substances that indicate bone loss. The advantage of this test is that it gives a dynamic picture of bone turnover and the rate of bone loss, rather than just a static single measure, as in the other tests.

There is also one simple test you can do yourself. For most of our life our height measures roughly the same as our arm span, from the tips of our fingers on our left hand to the tips of our fingers on our right. If we are suffering bone loss, our height will decline in relation to our arm span. So it's worth monitoring this measurement from time to time to see if there is any change.

Natural prevention of osteoporosis

As we have discovered, making sure we get enough calcium through food or supplements is only part of the picture. We have to make sure that we are not constantly depleting our supplies at the same time. And there are plenty of other ways we can help prevent osteoporosis.

1. **Exercise**   Regular exercise that makes an impact on our bones is crucial. These "weight-bearing" forms of exercise that actually build bone include dancing, walking, jogging, and bouncing. The importance of exercise in preventing osteoporosis has been widely ignored, largely because it is not in anyone's commercial interest to sell the idea to women or to conduct expensive research projects when there will be no "product" to promote at the end of it. One study showed that thirty women increased their spinal mass by 0.5 percent in one year with fifty minutes of vigorous walking four times a week while the non-exercisers lost 7 percent of their bone mass over the same period.[11] Weight-bearing exercise strengthens bones, increases bone mass, and increases the speed of your reactions, so reducing the chances of a bone-breaking fall.

2. **Get rid of aluminum pans**   Aluminum is a heavy toxic metal which enters the food through cooking. It interferes with the body's ability to metabolize calcium. The same applies to aluminum foil and containers. Use cast-iron, enamel, glass, and stainless-steel cookware instead. Avoid any coated cookware such as non-stick frying pans, which are believed to be carcinogenic.

3. **Increase your calcium absorption**   There is a simple way to do this. Take 15ml. (1 tablespoon) of cider vinegar and honey in a cupful of warm water up to three times a day. This drink helps you assimilate the calcium in your food and aids its absorption.

4. **Eat an alkaline diet**   The body calls on your calcium reserves to neutralize the food you eat. So it makes sense to ensure that you have a mainly alkaline diet. That way, your calcium is not continuously being leeched in order to correct an over-acid diet. Alkaline foods include all vegetables, fruits, sprouted seeds, yogurt, almonds, brazil nuts, and buckwheat, and they should form the bulk of our diet.

5. **Take care with tea**   If you drink tea with your meals, the tannin in it binds to important minerals and prevents their absorption in the digestive tract. Leave a gap of at least one hour before or after eating if you are going to have a cup of regular tea.

6. **Reduce stress in your life**   Stress, constant stress, is bad for bones. Most of us know that stress causes the release of adrenaline in the body. And too much adrenaline has a harmful dissolving effect on bone. Estrogen helps stimulate the liver to produce a protein that protects our bones against adrenaline. But by reducing stress in our lives and learning techniques to help us relax, we can reduce the amount of adrenaline being released in the first place. What is not often realized is that the food we eat has a huge impact on the amount of adrenaline released in the body. The wrong diet can cause internal stress, too. If you go too long without food, or have sugary foods, chocolate, tea, or coffee, your blood sugar level drops. This drop releases adrenaline into the bloodstream to boost your blood sugar level. We need to eat good-quality food little and often to maintain our blood sugar level.

7. **Beware of bran**   Bran has been hyped as a food that increases the amount of fiber in your diet. The reality is that it is a refined food containing substances called phytates which make certain vital nutrients like iron, zinc, and magnesium hard to absorb. Phytates also bind calcium, making it harder for your body to absorb this essential mineral. Don't sprinkle bran on your food or eat it in cereals where it is added as one of the main ingredients. It is better to eat bran in the form that nature intended—as part of a whole grain such as wheat. Raw

grains also contain phytates—so when you eat granola, for instance, you should soak it overnight to break them down. Granola can be soaked in water or juice.

8. **Keep an eye on your digestion** Low levels of stomach acid, more common as we get older, inhibit the absorption of calcium. There are numerous symptoms of low stomach acid, e.g. flatulence, bloating, indigestion, a feeling of fullness after eating, etc. If you experience any of these on a regular basis it may be worth having further investigations.

Supplements for osteoporosis

Calcium deficiency is only one of the factors believed to contribute to the onset of osteoporosis. Other vitamin and mineral deficiencies also play a part, along with caffeine and alcohol, falling hormone levels, smoking, digestive problems, and a sedentary way of life. But calcium is very important because it plays a major role in virtually every function of the body. The level of circulating calcium in your blood is so crucial that the body has a fail-safe mechanism to take calcium from your bones to keep the blood level constant. This is going on all the time. So it is not particularly helpful to assess your calcium levels through blood tests, since the level may be constantly changing. Calcium, with other minerals, forms your body skeleton. It also plays a part in the relaxation and contraction of your muscles—which is why people suffering from cramps are often told to take calcium supplements. And it affects your blood pressure, too. The more calcium you excrete, the more chance you have of raised blood pressure. This underlines once again the fact that the balance of calcium in the body is more important than just the amount you take.

FOOD CALCIUM CONTENT

Most of us have been brainwashed into believing that milk and other dairy products are the best sources of calcium,

Calcium content in various foods per 100g.

Milk	100mg.
Cheese	250–800mg.
Sesame seeds	630mg.
Almonds	282mg.
Sea vegetables (kelp)	400–1400mg.
Greens	140–160mg.
Sprats	710mg.
Haddock	100mg.
Broccoli	61mg.
Carrots	47mg.
Figs	280mg.

or that we need to take calcium supplements to stave off the threat of osteoporosis. The recommended daily intake of calcium is 500–1,000mg. As the table shows, it does not take much to reach that level. And there are plenty of calcium-rich foods besides dairy products.

While it is certainly true that milk and other dairy products contain high amounts of calcium, it is debatable whether this is the best and most effective way for human beings to get their dietary calcium. One interesting fact discovered by researchers was that breast-fed babies absorbed more calcium from their mothers' milk than from cows' milk despite the fact that cows' milk contains four times the amount of calcium. This underlines again the fact that the important thing is how the body uses the calcium— many people believe that our systems were not really designed to cope with cows' milk. A study of 1,000 women found that those who ate foods rich in potassium, magnesium, fiber and vitamin C—a high fruit and vegetable diet—had significantly higher bone density than those who had diets low in these nutrients. The conclusion was that fruit and vegetables were more likely to protect women against loss of bone mass and osteoporosis than milk and cheese. As we will see, these other nutrients play a vital role in putting calcium into our bones.

NOT ALL CALCIUM SUPPLEMENTS ARE EQUAL

We know that absorption of calcium is a crucial issue. When it comes to taking supplements, you should be aware that some are much more easily absorbed than others. Some are so poorly absorbed you are wasting your money—and possibly doing more harm than good. So when you buy supplements look very carefully at the labels. **Calcium carbonate** is one of the cheapest and most available forms of calcium supplement. It is otherwise known as chalk. It is an inorganic mineral, is mined from the ground, and is not present in this particular form in any plant or animal. It can increase the risk of kidney stones and chalky lumps in the breasts and can be deposited in the joints, contributing to arthritis. Its efficiency as a supplement is highly questionable, since research demonstrates that in this form calcium is not well absorbed into the system. Indeed there is some evidence that calcium carbonate supplements caused more calcium to be excreted in the urine when taken by women with adequate levels of stomach acid.[12] They might even have been losing more calcium than they were taking in. **Calcium citrate**, on the other hand, was found to be absorbed well even by women with low stomach acid. In one study, 500mg. of calcium citrate was absorbed better than even 2,000mg. of calcium carbonate.[13]

There is a confusing range of calcium supplements on the market. If you want to know how well the one you are taking is being absorbed, do the following test. Place your supplement in a glass of warm vinegar for thirty minutes, stirring every few minutes. The warm vinegar roughly represents the conditions found in your gut. If the supplement does not dissolve after half an hour, try another type.

MAGNESIUM

Magnesium is extremely important in bone health, equally, if not more important than calcium. Sixty percent of our body's magnesium stores are contained in our bones, particularly in the trabecular bone of the wrists, thighs, and vertebrae. It has been shown that women suffering from osteoporosis have lower levels of magnesium in their tra-becular bone than healthy women. This is not surprising because magnesium is vital in metabolizing calcium and vitamin C and helps to convert vitamin D to the active form necessary to ensure efficient calcium absorption. Magne-sium also activates the enzyme alkaline phosphatase. This enzyme helps to form calcium crystals in the bone and is often used as an indicator as to whether new bone is being formed. A study by Biolab in London compared different groups of women, some with osteoporosis, some postmen-opausal but with no osteoporosis, and some women on HRT.[14] They found that *none* of the women in any group had low levels of calcium. But the women with osteopo-rosis had low levels of other vital bone nutrients including magnesium and zinc, and of the enzyme alkaline phospha-tase, indicating poor bone renewal. A normal level of this enzyme is dependent on having enough magnesium in the body.

Magnesium also prevents the buildup of unwanted cal-cium deposits elsewhere in the body. We need *twice* as much magnesium as calcium if the biochemistry of bone formation is to run smoothly. Most of us, in fact, are mag-nesium deficient rather than calcium deficient. Good sources of dietary magnesium are dark green vegetables, apples, seeds, nuts, figs, and lemons. The importance of magnesium in the bone-building process has been demon-strated. In one research project two groups of women were monitored. One group took HRT plus magnesium. The other took HRT alone. After nine months the bone mineral density of the women taking magnesium had increased by 11 percent. The women taking only HRT showed no in-crease in bone mineral density. After two years the mag-nesium takers were still improving their bone density.[15]

VITAMIN C

Vitamin C is crucial for bone formation. Its chief function here is to produce collagen, which makes up some 90 per-cent of our bone matrix. Collagen is also important for the growth and repair of cells, gums, blood vessels, and teeth. We do not manufacture our own vitamin C. We rely on what we eat and drink. We don't store it, either. Vitamin C is water soluble and excreted within two or three hours, so we need to get adequate amounts daily. Good sources are citrus fruits, green and leafy vegetables, cauliflower, berries, potatoes, and sweet potatoes.

VITAMIN D

This vitamin is fat soluble, unlike vitamin C, and is acquired through sunlight or diet. It helps the vital absorption of calcium and phosphorus from the digestive process and helps put them into bone. A deficiency of vitamin D leads to decalcification of bones. Good sources are fish and fish oils.

ZINC

This important mineral helps the activity of vitamin D in promoting calcium absorption. Osteoporosis sufferers are frequently low in zinc. Good sources are oysters, fish, animal foods, pumpkin seeds, and eggs.

PHOSPHORUS

We need some phosphorus to help make bone. But most of us have far too much of it, which upsets the calcium chemistry in the body. Excess phosphorus in the bloodstream sends a message that more calcium is required, and stores are released from the bones. Some scientists believe that getting the calcium/phosphorus ratio right is more important than calcium alone in protecting bones. Nowadays it's very easy to consume far too much phosphorus. It's there in all kinds of food—instant soups and desserts, meat, cheese, toppings, cola drinks, and other carbonated beverages. Cut down on all of these. The ideal balance is equal parts of calcium to phosphorus. But research suggests we consume four times as much phosphorus as calcium. Cottage cheese, for example, contains far more phosphorus than calcium.

BORON

Some minerals—phosphorus, calcium, and magnesium, for instance—are termed macro minerals because they are present in our bodies in large amounts. Zinc, manganese, copper, chromium, selenium, and boron, on the other hand, are present in small amounts and are known as trace elements. Boron is in fact an "ultratrace" element—the amounts needed are even smaller. But boron is now believed to be vital for a number of reasons. A U.S. Department of Agriculture research study demonstrated that giving postmenopausal women a short course of 3mg. boron supplements a day resulted in a 44 percent reduction in the amount of calcium excreted in their urine.[15] It also markedly increased the amount of the estrogen hormone estradiol in their blood. In fact it raised the level of this estrogen to the amounts shown in the blood of women receiving estrogen therapy. The conclusions of this rather dramatic Department of Agriculture study were that boron improved the metabolism of calcium, phosphorus, and magnesium, helped raise estrogen levels in older women to the levels found in those taking HRT, helped in the manufacture of vitamin D needed for calcium absorption, and reduced calcium, magnesium, and estrogen loss. Boron is found in alfalfa, kelp, cabbage, and leafy greens. It is stored in our bones and any excess is excreted in the urine.

VITAMIN B6

Diets deficient in vitamin B6 have produced osteoporosis in rats.[15] It appears to increase the strength of connective tissue in bone. You can find vitamin B6 in everyday foods such as whole grains, fish, nuts, bananas, and avocados.

VITAMIN K

Vitamin K is known primarily for its effect on blood clotting. But it is also needed to synthesize osteocalcin, a unique protein found in large amounts in bone. Osteocalcin helps harden calcium, so vitamin K is vital for bone formation. In one study of sixteen osteoporosis patients, blood levels of vitamin K were found to be 35 percent lower than in healthy people of the same age.[16] Frequent use of antibiotics can result in vitamin K deficiency. The best source of vitamin K is green vegetables.

Homeopathy and osteoporosis

A homeopath treats a menopausal patient by giving an appropriate constitutional remedy, taking into account any other symptoms of the menopause. Often the homeopathic remedy Calcarea phosphoricum (Cal phos) is recommended, especially for fair-skinned, tall, thin women who are believed to be at a higher risk of bone loss. If you are not tall and thin, take Calcarea carbonicum (Calc carb) 6X potency three times a day.

Herbal medicine and osteoporosis

In herbal medicine some remedies are chosen for their calcium content, while other remedies will help to balance hormones. Herbs such as horsetail (equisetum) and alfalfa are often used for the long-term treatment of osteoporosis.

Reducing the risk factors

Whatever your lifestyle has been up till now, it is never too late to make changes. Your body is extraordinarily resilient, and given the chance it will work to restore health and get your hormones back in balance. You can reduce obvious risk factors by giving up smoking and lowering your intake of tea, coffee, and alcohol. You can start taking exercise more seriously. More importantly, you should now be able to see that the food you eat is the vitally important first line of defense against bone loss. On this, all the complex biochemical processes of bone formation and maintenance depend. Osteoporosis is still only imperfectly understood— even by the medical experts. As the British National Osteoporosis Society states, "Lack of research into osteoporosis means we don't know all the answers to treating this disease, so prevention is vital." Bone loss and osteoporosis are not inevitable as we age. A 1993 study by the Metabolic Bone Disease Center in Italy found that many women maintained their bone density for thirty to forty years after the menopause.[17] There is now plenty of evidence that our diets and the nutrients they contain (or lack) are crucial factors in bone loss and its prevention. In time, osteoporosis may be seen as a lifestyle disorder rather than a menopausal "problem." Meanwhile, there is plenty you can do to protect yourself. The choice is yours.

What to do

What would be a good all-around supplement program to give you the best protection against osteoporosis, remembering that you also need to look after your diet and exercise?

1. Eat a good whole food diet with a wide variety of fresh fruit and vegetables. The more variety you have, the greater your chance of getting the vitamins and minerals you need from your food. Keep protein content low, and eliminate or reduce caffeine.
2. Design a convenient exercise schedule for yourself to follow.
3. Buy a good multivitamin and mineral supplement for the menopause which contains boron, such as New Chapter, New Spirit Natural, Vita Balance 2000, or Rainbow Light.

Add the following supplements:
- Vitamin C—1,000mg. three times per day
- Zinc Citrate—15mg. per day
- A combined magnesium and calcium supplement with no more than 500mg. of calcium citrate per day
- Vitamin B complex—50mg. per day
- Linseed oil—1,000mg. once per day.

CHAPTER 8

Your breasts at the menopause

Fear of breast cancer is very real for many women. And the United States has one of the highest rates of breast cancer in the world. The disease is the leading cause of death among American women between the ages of 15 and 54, and about 44,000 women of all ages die from it here each year. Most of us know someone who has had breast cancer and endured what can be traumatic treatment. Many of us would admit it is our biggest dread. And as we get older, the statistical chances of developing breast cancer increase. The best approach to protecting yourself is to be armed with information. This chapter gives you that information and lays out what choices are available to help you protect your breasts.

No one knows for certain what causes breast cancer. Overweight, excess consumption of saturated fats, alcohol, emotional distress, family history, exposure to pesticides and radiation, and the hormonal changes of the menopause have all been linked to it, but no conclusive cause has emerged. However, research does indicate that some women seem to be more at risk than others. These women may have a mother or sister who has had breast cancer. Obese women, those who have never had children, and women who gave birth for the first time after the age of thirty-five seem to have a higher risk, as do women who started their periods early and had a late menopause. Other factors include starting the Pill at a very young age and staying on it for more than four years and also not breast-feeding babies. A small minority of breast cancer cases, about 10 percent, seem to be linked to inheriting a faulty gene called BRAC 1. And women do seem to run higher

146

risks of breast cancer at and after the menopause. The table on page 148 shows how breast cancer risk for women goes up with age.

Yet these statistics are not universal. In some parts of the world, notably the Far East, breast cancer is not the major killer it is here in the West. Why? The United States has a breast cancer death rate that is several times higher than that of women in Japan, for instance, which gives us an important clue. Studies conducted in the United States have shown that when Japanese women move to the West, they are more likely to develop breast cancer.[1] The level then rises to one similar to that seen here. Many experts think the main factor is diet, and this is borne out by the fact that as the traditional Japanese diet becomes more Westernized, cases of breast cancer are increasing among Japanese women in Japan itself.

There are a number of differences between the normal Japanese diet and ours. They eat a good quantity of unsaturated fats in oils and fish, whereas the Western diet is high in saturated fat from meat and dairy foods. The traditional Japanese do not eat much dairy food at all. The other main difference is their large consumption of soybean products including tofu, miso (soybean paste), tamari (wheat-free soy sauce), tempeh, and soy milk. What currently fascinates cancer researchers is the idea that it is something in this diet that has protected the Japanese from certain kinds of cancers by maintaining the balance between normal healthy cell development and the over-multiplication of cells that is the first detectable sign of cancer. Changing your diet may be the best way to protect yourself from breast cancer.

The process that makes a cell cancerous is the same process by which a cell grows and replicates. With cancer, the cells seem to be doing the job too well. The control mechanism that would normally stop a cell from multiplying seems to be at fault. The multiplication seems to continue with no controls. It is interesting that this overgrowth and multiplication can be happening all over our bodies at different times and yet does not necessarily produce cancer. When our cells are functioning well and our immune system is good, cancer does not develop.

Breast cancer risk	
Age	Risk in next ten years
20	1 in 2,500
30	1 in 233
40	1 in 65
50	1 in 41
60	1 in 29

Source: The American Cancer Society

Surgery to remove cancerous growths is based on the assumption that these tumors are separate, independent manifestations of the disease that are unconnected to the general health of the rest of the body and that removal of the diseased part, if caught in time, can prevent the cancer from spreading. Surgery removes as much of the cancer as possible but does not address the underlying cause. So although that one lump may have been removed, cancer may reappear at another site because the factors that caused the cancer in the first place are still there. This theory is supported by recent research involving 5,500 breast cancer patients—one of the largest investigations of its kind. It demonstrated that mastectomy (radical surgery involving the removal of breast tissue and all lymph nodes in the armpit) guaranteed women no greater survival rates than if they had a lumpectomy (lump only removed) and radiation.[2]

Modern medicine, in many cases, focuses on treating the symptoms rather than the cause. A good metaphor is the one in which the hardworking doctors are busy mopping up the floor covered with water which is overspilling from the sink above, where both faucets are on full and the plug is in. They are frantically treating the never ending ''symptom,'' whereas the natural treatment would be to find and remove the cause—i.e., take out the plug and turn off the faucets.

Breast tenderness and lumps are known to respond to an

increased intake of essential fatty acids, so these oils should be an important part of our diet both for prevention and treatment. And a very interesting study in the British *Journal of Nutrition* showed that soybeans can have a balancing effect on the estrogen in our bodies.[3] The soy increased estrogen levels when they were low and reduced them when they were too high. It seems to explain why soybeans can reduce hot flashes (which are thought to be due to a lack of estrogen) and also reduce the incidence of breast cancer (which is thought to be linked to an excess of the hormone). Increasingly researchers believe that some constituents found in certain foods, like soy, which forms an important part of traditional Japanese and other Eastern diets, effectively protect women from hormonally linked cancers.

Most breast problems are benign, not cancerous. Many women complain of tender, swollen breasts and lumps that fluctuate with the menstrual cycle—fibrocystic breasts. These can be so painful that the women's lives are seriously affected. Some women can't bear to hug their children and cannot bear to be hugged by their partners. It can make sexual intercourse uncomfortable. Other women can't wear tight clothing, and some have difficulty sleeping because they can't find a comfortable position. In extreme cases some women have opted for mastectomies.

But fibrocystic breasts can be helped with nutrition. This can be done by avoiding drinks that contain methylxanthines (coffee, tea, chocolate, cola, and even decaffeinated coffee), as these have been shown to cause breast tenderness. Follow the recommendations in Chapter 6 on Natural Alternatives to HRT (see page 96), and increase the intake of essential fatty acids in your food by eating plenty of oily fish, nuts, and seeds. Add in some supplements containing oils such as evening primrose oil, linseed oil, or fish oils.

Be breast aware

You need to become familiar with the shape of your breasts. You need to know their appearance and how they feel. Then you will notice if anything starts to change.

Spend time looking at them in the mirror, perhaps when undressing for bed or before getting into the bath or shower.

CHECK THEM OUT

1. Stand in front of the mirror, raise your arms above your head, and move from side to side to get a good look at your breasts. Get to know how they feel and look at the shape and outline. Become aware of the position and shape of the nipple.
2. Lie on your back with your head on a pillow. Examine one breast at a time. Raise your right arm and put it behind your head. Using the tips of your left fingers, feel around the right breast in small circular movements. Check both breasts and armpits in the same way.

What to look for:

1. Any small lump in the breast or armpit.
2. A dimple or dent in the skin when lifting your arm.
3. Any reddish, ulcerated, or scaly area of skin on the breast or nipple.
4. Any bleeding or discharge from the nipple or moist, reddish areas that don't heal easily.
5. Any change in nipple position—i.e. pulled inward or pointing in a different direction.

If you are concerned about anything you find, you should consult your doctor immediately. More than 90 percent of breast tumors are first detected by women themselves, including some cancers that can be felt but go undetected by a mammogram.

UNDERSTAND THE ROLE OF ESTROGEN

Estrogen's role in the body is as a ''builder,'' helping to build the lining of the womb ready to receive a fertilized egg during every menstrual cycle. You can see logically that increased cell growth could lead to cancer. The use of estrogens and HRT has been linked to an increased risk of breast cancer in a number of studies. It has been estimated that the risk of breast cancer increases by 15 to 30 percent after ten years of estrogen therapy.[4] It would also explain why women who have a surgical menopause seem to suffer less breast cancer (less estrogen circulating) and why women who start their periods early and have a late menopause have a higher risk (more estrogen present for a greater number of years).

A fascinating study reported in the September 1994 edition of the *Journal of the National Cancer Institute* showed that women who exercised for around four hours a week had a 58 percent lower risk of breast cancer and those who routinely exercised for between one and three hours a week had a 30 percent lower risk.[5] This investigation compared two groups of women under the age of forty and concluded that their activity patterns were a significant predictor of breast cancer risk. What the researchers did not know was precisely why. The thinking is that regular exercise modifies a woman's hormonal activity in a beneficial way. We know that extremes of exercise alter the menstrual cycle dramatically—many women athletes, for instance, don't have periods at all. So the suggestion is that moderate routine exercise suppresses the production (or overproduction) of hormones, reducing a woman's exposure during her lifetime. As the researchers pointed out, this highlighted one real way that women could protect themselves from adolescence onward. And it supports the belief that estrogen may be implicated in breast cancer. Establishing lifetime exercise routines is important before, through, and after the menopause to reduce the risk of breast cancer.

Obviously we can choose not to take HRT if we think it poses an unacceptable risk. Unfortunately, we are also bombarded from estrogens in the environment. These are called xenoestrogens (foreign estrogens). In an article in *Environmental Health Perspectives* entitled "Medical Hypothesis: Xenoestrogens, a preventable cause of breast cancer," the authors put forward the theory that we are becoming engulfed in these foreign estrogens from a number of different sources.[6] Pesticides sprayed on crops are a major source of xenoestrogens, and they are also found in plastics. One, in particular, is the chemical bisphenol A, which is a byproduct of the plastics industry. The fact that bisphenol A produces estrogenic effects in humans became alarmingly clear when some men working in the plastics industry developed breasts after inhaling the chemical in dust. We can absorb these chemicals into our bodies by putting our food in plastic containers or by buying sandwiches, fruit, and vegetables, etc. with plastic coverings. The same is true for drinks in plastic bottles or cooking food in the microwave.

Just how potent these xenoestrogens are was discovered by a group of scientists who found that alligators that had hatched in Lake Apopka, Florida, had abnormally small penises and altered hormone levels. They found that in 1980 there had been a massive spill of Kelthane, a pesticide, into the lake. The xenoestrogens from the pesticide were feminizing the alligators. The impact of xenoestrogen pollution has been seen elsewhere, too. Fish-eating birds in the Great Lakes region that had been contaminated by chlorinated organic compounds had an abnormally high rate of embryo deaths and deformities and unusual nesting behavior. Hundreds of these organo-chlorines have been shown to cause cancer in laboratory animals and humans. Some have been identified in breast cancers and have been banned or restricted, but many remain in everyday use. A few examples are the herbicide atrazine, vinyl chloride (used in vinyl-coated fabric), and methylene chloride (used in paint strippers). Women exposed to higher-than-normal levels of synthetic chemicals, through their jobs or through living near hazardous waste sites, have significantly higher rates of breast cancer. Women with the highest concentration of certain organo-chlorine pesticides in their bodies are at a higher risk of breast cancer than women with lower levels.

It's likely that these xenoestrogens get into the body to act on breast cells through fatty tissue. Synthetic estrogens tend to accumulate in fatty tissue. And, of course, this problem runs right through the food chain. Food from animals is likely to contain larger doses of xenoestrogens than food from other organisms. So meat from animals that eat smaller animals or contaminated grass, grain, or water is likely to give more exposure than a plate of vegetables that have been sprayed with pesticides.

Until recently women were officially advised to examine themselves for any changes in their breasts. Then in 1991, the medical officer at the British Department of Health stated that self-examination had not resulted in a fall in mortality rates. This obviously caused a shock among health advisers and women themselves. To lessen the damage of this remark, the British government then changed its position to suggest that women should be "breast aware," meaning aware of anything that seemed unusual in their breasts.

Benefits and risks of mammography

A mammogram is a breast X-ray, and although it is commonly recommended to detect breast cancer it has its negative side. First, X-rays can cause breast cancer, so ironically you could be exposing yourself to a test that can trigger the disease it is supposed to be detecting. Second, mammography can result in false readings. These false-positives mean that women may be recalled to have another mammogram and another dose of X-rays, not to mention the emotional stress and anxiety the diagnosis causes.

There have been warnings about mammograms since the early 1980s when the late Dr. Robert Mendelsohn published a book, *Male Practice, How Doctors Manipulate Women*. He warned that annual screening of women who had no symptoms might well produce more cancer than it detects. This unfortunately was borne out quite dramatically in a Canadian study in 1989, where the National Breast Screening Trial examined more than 89,000 women between the ages of forty and forty-nine over an eight-year period.[7] Half the women in the group received mammograms every year. The researchers found that these women had a significantly higher death rate than those in the other half of the group, who had not been given a mammogram. The women who had the mammograms had a 52 percent increase in deaths from breast cancer.

The excellent regular British publication *What Doctors Don't Tell You* (*WDDTY*) has published a guide to women's screening tests which has a very informative section on mammograms. It suggests that if you decide to have a mammogram you should do some homework. It gives a four-point check list:

1. Is the equipment used specifically designed for mammograms? This is important because it means the equipment can give the best image with the least radiation.
2. How many mammograms are done at this facility? *WDDTY* quotes the American College of Radiology, which recommends going to a lab or hospital where each radiologist reads at least ten mammograms a week. Obviously this will reduce the number of false readings.
3. When was the machine last inspected and calibrated to check it is giving out the intended dose of radiation? It should be checked once a year.
4. How old is the equipment?

Other safer tests in the pipeline are the transillumination test with infrared light scanning, in which a light is shone on the breast and lumps show up by blocking the light. The antimalignane antibody serum (AMAS) test measures serum levels of AMA, an antibody found in higher amounts in most patients in the early stages of active non-terminal malignancies.

The wait-and-see approach

It may be beneficial to get a second opinion if you have been diagnosed with a breast lump or cancer and treatment has been offered. An interesting report in *The Lancet* in 1992 stated that many small cancers would have remained dormant if left undiscovered, according to findings at postmortems. Sometimes the wait-and-see approach can be useful, but you need a medical doctor with a conservative attitude to breast problems. A woman who came to see me for help with her menopausal symptoms told me that years before, she had found a breast lump which her consultant said he would leave but monitor. That was ten years ago, and the breast lump has now gone.

Can your clothing affect your breasts?

An interesting book entitled *Dressed to Kill* suggests that wearing a bra can increase the risk of breast cancer by suppressing the lymphatic system, causing toxins to accumulate in the breasts.[8] I found the concept interesting. The connection between clothing and disease has been noticed before. The kind of tight corsets worn by women in the late nineteenth and early twentieth centuries, which really constricted the waist, were associated with high rates of heart, liver, and kidney problems. More recently, male infertility and possible testicular cancer has been linked to men's wearing tight underpants. It is our lymphatic system that filters toxins and accumulated waste from our blood. Anything that stops the flow of lymph, such as tight clothing, like a bra, can indeed cause an accumulation of these toxins.

The statistics from the bra study showed that women who wore a bra for more than twelve hours a day were more likely to develop breast cancer than those who wore their bras for a shorter time. Because this study was flawed in strict scientific terms, it is unwise to place too much emphasis on its results. But I think that sensibly we should give our breasts a chance to "breathe." Try not to sleep in your bra, and try to get loose-fitting cotton nightwear that does not constrict your breasts. Choose a bra made of natural fibers like cotton, so that at least your breasts can breathe through the natural fiber rather than being trapped inside nylon.

Make sure you have a properly fitting bra. This can make a difference to your posture (badly fitting bras can result in shoulder and neck pain) and breast tenderness. To find your correct size: measure around your rib cage in inches and add 4 to an odd number or 5 to an even one. To find your cup size: measure around your breasts at the fullest part and subtract this rib cage measurement from the breast measurement. A difference of:

0 in.	(0cm.)	=	A cup
1 in.	(2.5cm.)+	=	B cup
2 in.	(5.0cm.)+	=	C cup
3 in.	(7.5cm.)+	=	D cup
4 in.	(10cm.)+	=	DD cup
5 in.	(13cm.)+	=	E cup

PREVENTING BREAST CANCER

As in all things, prevention is better than cure. If you can keep yourself in optimum health, you give your body a better chance to keep the multiplication of cells under control. Cells have to multiply to grow and rejuvenate. We would die if that did not happen. But again, there is the importance of balance. Cells multiply for healthy reasons, but when they overmultiply it can lead to cancer. A healthy body has a better chance of keeping the balance.

Scientists have now found that major crises such as bereavement, job loss, and divorce are associated with breast cancer. A team of researchers from Taiwan's National Chen Kung University Medical College questioned 199 women aged between twenty and seventy who had been recalled to London's King's College Hospital with a suspicious breast lump or abnormality. They found that the risk of developing breast cancer increased by three to four times if the woman had suffered severe stress in the previous five years. Fascinatingly, the researchers discovered that women who had confronted their problems and tried to work them out were three times more likely to suffer breast cancer than those who had expressed their emotions and become very upset. Perhaps the ability to let go and be upset is a kind of emotional and physical release. Just being postmenopausal did not seem to be an important risk factor in this study.

Taking an active role in actually trying to prevent breast cancer is important in our society, where we are bombarded with environmental factors from many different sources.

We can help ourselves by maintaining a strong and healthy immune system so that the growth and repair of cells is kept in check. The foods we eat can strengthen our immune system. We can avoid foods that weaken it. And we can also take steps at home to reduce the level of toxins we are exposed to. Diet is absolutely crucial, since up to 60 percent of all cancers are believed to be linked to diet and nutrition.[9]

EAT THE RIGHT KIND OF FAT

A number of studies in respected journals, such as the *New England Journal of Medicine*, have looked at the connection between dietary fat and risk of breast cancer. In 1988, the U.S. Surgeon General stated that the top priority in the prevention of chronic diseases, including cancer, was the reduction of dietary fat. By this he meant saturated fat in the form found in animals' milk, cheese, and red meat, not the unsaturated fats found in oils, nuts, seeds, and fish, which seem to have a protective effect especially against breast cancer. A study reported in the *Journal of the National Cancer Institute* in 1995 showed that olive oil in the diet lowered the risk of breast cancer.[10]

ENJOY A HEALTHY GENERAL DIET

Cancer rates are lower in people who eat the most fruits and vegetables. Cruciferous vegetables such as cabbage, broccoli, and brussels sprouts help to guard against cancer because they contain the compound indol-3-carbinol, which changes the way estrogen is metabolized in the body.

The more antioxidant-rich foods we eat, the more protection it seems to give. Diets high in beta-carotene—found in carrots, sweet potatoes, and dark green leafy vegetables such as kale and Swiss chard—have been shown to protect against cancer. In a study conducted at Harvard University, beta-carotene altered the proteins needed for tumors to grow. Citrus fruits, with their powerful mix of natural substances, including carotenoids and flavonoids, have been shown to neutralize powerful chemical carcinogens in animals.

Antioxidants include vitamin A (in the form of beta-carotene), vitamin E, vitamin C, and selenium. Low levels of selenium have been directly linked to higher rates of cancer.

Allium vegetables, which include garlic, onions, and scallions, have been found to contain certain cancer-inhibiting properties. Garlic's sulfur compounds increase the activity of macrophages and T-lymphocytes, two components of the immune system that destroy tumor cells.

EAT PHYTOESTROGENS

Phytoestrogens are a group of foods that contain substances that have a hormone-like action. Soybeans, for instance, contain phyto-chemicals known as isoflavones which make up about 75 percent of the soy protein. In the human gut, bacteria convert isoflavones into compounds that can have an estrogenic action, although they are not hormones. These phyto-estrogens seem to fit into estrogen receptors on breast cancer cells but are probably too weak to stimulate the cells. What seems to happen is that these weak estrogens block the estrogen receptors and prevent cancer from developing.[11] In simple terms, they prevent the estrogens in the body from latching on. The two flavonoid compounds, genistein and daidzein, that have this mild estrogenic activity also help to reduce cholesterol.[12]

Soybeans have been found to contain at least five compounds believed to inhibit cancer. One of these compounds is chemically similar to the drug Tamoxifen, which is now used to treat estrogen-dependent breast cancer. Tamoxifen works as an estrogen receptor antagonist: that is, it binds on to the estrogen receptors and inhibits cancer growth. Tests show that the Japanese, for example, have high levels of isoflavones in their urine and plasma—much higher than the amount found among the Americans and British—indicating that their traditional diet supplies them naturally with the phyto-estrogens that may prevent hormonally linked cancers. Japanese women have been shown to excrete phyto-estrogens in their urine 100–1,000 times higher than those excreted by American women.[13] The good news for the rest of us is that one research project, reported in the *British Medical Journal* in 1993, demonstrated that concentrations of daidzein and other isoflavones in plasma could be easily and quickly raised by foods (in this case soy, clover sprouts, and linseed) containing phyto-estrogens.[14]

Other examples of foods that contain phyto-estrogens are whole grains, legumes (such as chickpeas, lentils, garlic, and peas), fennel, celery, parsley, rhubarb, and hops.

INCREASE YOUR FIBER INTAKE

Fiber is very important because it determines how much estrogen we store and how much we excrete. Soluble fiber binds estrogen so that it is excreted more efficiently. Chronic constipation has been linked to breast cancer. That's not surprising, because toxic waste products that are not dealt with properly can end up stored in the body's fatty tissue, including the breasts. The importance of fiber as far as breast cancer is concerned has not been adequately stressed.

Women worried about breast cancer are often told to watch their intake of fat—which is good general health advice. What is not pointed out is that the fiber factor—increasing the amount of fruit and vegetables in your diet—seems to be much more important in prevention.

AVOID ENVIRONMENTAL TOXINS WHERE POSSIBLE

This is really a case of do the best you can, because you cannot control everything. Use filtered water to reduce your intake of chlorine and lead by using either an under-the-sink filter or a simple pitcher filter.

Buy organic vegetables and grains where possible to eliminate your intake of pesticides. Also try to avoid using pesticides yourself in the garden, and see if you can find other more environmentally friendly ways to control pests, such as putting certain plants together.

Take a look at the cosmetics, toiletries, and deodorants you use, and try to buy those that contain the most natural ingredients. Even though products may include only small amounts of chemicals, it is the cumulative and cocktail effect that may cause problems. Many deodorants contain aluminum, a heavy toxic metal, so buy an aluminum-free one from a health food store. Ask for white fillings instead of mercury amalgams at the dentist.

Use products containing the smallest amount of chemicals to clean your house and your clothes so that you are not filling your home environment with unwanted toxins.

Try to buy fruit and vegetables loose, so that they are not wrapped tightly in plastic. At home, avoid using plastic wrap and storing food for long periods in plastic containers. In the fridge you can just use glass dishes with lids to store food. You are not going to be able to prevent all your food from coming into contact with plastic, because that is the nature of our society. Just do the best you can where it is in your control.

Women often feel helpless in the face of what appears to be a rising tide of breast cancer. As we get older, more of our friends and relatives seem to become victims. But I hope I have shown that there is a great deal that you can do in terms of prevention, both for yourself and for your daughters. The major research studies on the subject, some of which I have mentioned here, reveal that diet is absolutely crucial, that what we eat is as important as what we avoid. It lies within the power of all of us to use what is already known in our own daily lives. We can do something positive, and we should.

CHAPTER 9

Your heart at the menopause

Increasingly women are told they should take HRT to protect themselves from heart attacks. It is true that as we get older our pattern of heart attack risk changes. Between the ages of thirty-five and forty-four, for instance, we have a six times lower risk of cardiovascular disease than men of the same age. But by the time we are fifty, we have half as much risk of heart disease. It is not until we get to the age of seventy-five that we have an equal risk to men. So what causes us to lose our protection? It has been assumed that because estrogen levels drop at the menopause it's this that puts us at a higher risk of heart attacks. Estrogen is thought to have a beneficial effect on blood cholesterol metabolism, so when levels fall we lose our advantage. This is an incredible assumption to make when there are so many other factors to be taken into account in heart disease. There has been an overwhelming amount of research conducted on men and heart disease but comparatively little is known about heart disease in women. The famous ongoing Framingham Study, which started in 1948 and follows the health of men and women in the United States, recently published in the *Journal of the American Medical Association* the results of a survey looking at the risk factors for heart attacks. Both men and women were included in this survey, but the researchers found that so few women suffered heart attacks that their results were not considered significant.[1]

When researchers tried to test out the theory that estrogen protects against heart disease, by giving men estrogen to see if it prevented a second heart attack, the study had to be halted because of the dramatic increase in heart attacks among the men given the hormone.[2] Perhaps that says it all.

This chapter will examine this whole area of HRT and heart disease, at the end of which the question may be asked, "What is the point of taking such a powerful drug with the real risk of side effects for a condition in which women have a low risk factor?"

Just where did the idea come from that HRT could prevent heart problems? The history of this rather dubious claim, which is incessantly repeated in media reports on the benefits of HRT, illustrates only too well an old adage of Winston Churchill's that there are lies, damn lies, and then there are statistics. The study that started all this off was reported in the *New England Journal of Medicine* in 1985, with a follow-up in 1991. It looked at data received from questionnaires sent out to 121,700 nurses every two years over a period of ten years. Eventually the study was reduced to 48,470 postmenopausal women.[3]

Every two years the questionnaires were sent out, and the nurses filled in the details of their food and alcohol intake over that two-year period. This required a great deal of motivation from the nurses to keep accurate records over such a long time.

More to the point was the way the research program was structured. Normally one group of women is randomly split into two groups, one group would be given HRT and the other a placebo (dummy pill). Then the women's progress would be followed over a number of years to study the comparative risk of heart disease. But this is not what happened with the nurses' study. There was no random selection of the groups in this case. One group was selected because they were already taking HRT and the other group was selected because they were not taking HRT.

It is very likely that those nurses who were at "high risk," who had a history of heart disease or knew it was in their family would probably not have been prescribed HRT in the first place. The researchers actually found that in the group not on HRT there were 29.5 percent more cigarette smokers and 29.6 percent more diabetics, who could be assumed to be at a higher risk of heart attacks anyway. So there was what researchers call a "selection bias." The results came out indicating that women on HRT had a lower risk of heart disease. In this experiment it is likely only the healthiest nurses with a low risk of heart disease would be in the group taking HRT. Those at a higher risk of heart attack would, by definition, not be taking HRT. This is not the same thing as demonstrating that HRT protects against heart disease. Not by a long way. But it is the simplistic message that makes the headlines. And the HRT industry is only too happy to reinforce it.

So we can't draw any firm conclusions from this study at all. Nor from the results of other U.S. studies which appear to show that women on HRT have a lower risk of heart disease. In the United States, the women who take HRT are usually middle class, health conscious, and comfortably off. They are likely to have less heart disease anyway. In fact in the very same issue of the *New England Journal of Medicine* that featured the nurses' study mentioned above were details of another study showing that use of estrogen substantially *increased* both heart disease and strokes,[4] and a review of a number of separate studies in *The Lancet* in 1991 concluded that the evidence for the preventive role of HRT in heart disease was either biased or insubstantial.

It also emerged that of the 48,470 menopausal women taking part in the study only 112 died of heart disease. That was 0.2 percent of the total—far too small a sample to yield any worthwhile conclusions as to the preventive effect of HRT. Yet it was claimed that taking estrogen had more than halved the risk of dying from heart disease. In fact nine out of ten of the nurses who died during the study succumbed to something other than heart disease.

This then is the basis of the claim, endorsed by some authorities in Britain over the last few years, that taking HRT *might* reduce heart disease by 50 percent. Amazingly, this claim became common currency, despite the fact that up to 1991, published results of research (done mostly in the U.S.) were based on estrogen only (unopposed HRT). From 1975 onward, with the scare about womb cancer, women in Britain have been given estrogen plus progestogen (opposed HRT). Nowadays opposed HRT is the most commonly prescribed form of HRT. Until the results of a follow-up survey were completed in 1992—not published until the summer of 1996—no one knew what the impact of added progestogen would be.[5] Yet the confident message broadcast for years before was that HRT could prevent heart disease. Here is the conclusion of the published results: "The addition of progestogen does not appear to attenuate the cardioprotective effects of postmenopausal estrogen therapy." In plain English, it is saying that adding progestogen to the estrogen does not appear to weaken the protective effects the estrogen has on the heart. But as we have seen from the above, it is far from conclusive that estrogen has any such protective effects. In fact, there are studies that show the reverse is true. A letter published in the *New England Journal of Medicine* in 1992 cited sixteen references that negated the claim that estrogen can be protective against cardiovascular disease.[6]

Other studies also seem to disprove the theory that estrogen levels have much to do with heart attack risk. One recent study reported in *The British Medical Journal* in 1995 investigated the link between individual women's own natural levels of estrogen and their risk of heart disease.[7] If the theory that estrogen supplementation protects against heart disease is correct, it would be logical to assume that women with relatively high levels of estrogen already in their bodies are at less risk of heart problems. The scientists studied 651 women, before and after the menopause, over a period of nineteen years, taking regular blood samples. They could establish no clear link between natural estrogen levels and heart disease. They observed that death rates from heart disease did not change at the age of fifty and concluded that the different levels of estrogen in pre- and postmenopausal women had nothing to do with the risk of heart problems, which suggests that estrogen supplementation at the menopause is of doubtful help for prevention.

For most women hormone levels at the menopause reduce very gradually; for others there is a more dramatic change. At the moment there is no routine blood testing, even for those women who are prescribed HRT. I have seen women who have had a total hysterectomy (ovaries removed too) and then automatically been given a hormone implant. One woman later found she had 2.5 times the normal level of estrogen in her blood. Were her estrogen levels normal before she was given the implant? And would it have been more appropriate to monitor those levels before hormones were given? She is now being tested regularly, as the HRT has been stopped, but her estrogen levels are still too high. Our hormones do fluctuate, even after the menopause, but a hormone profile may still be worthwhile.

Until more is known about this, it is clearly wrong to assume, as the advocates of HRT tend to do, that hormone deficiencies are the prime cause of all the symptoms and risks of the menopause.

So just what are the other factors that could give women an increased risk of heart disease beyond the menopause if the menopause itself and falling estrogen levels are not to blame?

A pathologist named Jerome Sullivan in South Carolina, posed the question why more men than women died from heart disease. He knew the prevailing theory was that estrogen was protecting women, but he had observed that women who had had a hysterectomy but kept their ovaries (which produce estrogen) had a higher risk of heart problems. He asked himself what the difference was. He realized that women who have had a hysterectomy and postmenopausal women don't have periods. Why would this make such a difference?

When we menstruate we lose about 500mg. of stored iron (ferritin) a year. Iron is a strange mineral. Until recently scientists thought the more iron we had, the better. Our bodies need iron to make red blood cells and to transport oxygen around the body. Without iron, new cells could not be produced, and our organs would be starved of oxygen. The negative side is that we do not eliminate iron; it is continually stored as ferritin. The only time we lose iron is during a period, childbirth, an accident occasioning blood loss, or by donating blood. Sullivan found that by the age of forty-five a man has as much iron in his blood as the average woman of seventy. At these ages men and women share the same statistical risk of heart attack. They also have similar average amounts of ferritin in their blood. This, rather than estrogen, might be the vital factor.

Jerome Sullivan published his findings connecting iron and heart disease in *The Lancet* in 1981, but the medical community was not impressed. They were still locked into producing drugs to lower cholesterol. It wasn't until 1990 that a cardiologist named John Murray, who had been studying nomadic African cattle herders, realized that even though their diet was mainly whole milk, high in saturated fat and cholesterol, none of the men over fifty had heart disease. Whole milk is low in iron, so Murray proposed that cholesterol is "bad" only when in the presence of iron's oxidizing effects. He decided to measure cholesterol's "stickiness" by giving the cattle herders extra iron for sixty days and found that when he did so, more of the "bad" cholesterol (LDL cholesterol; see below) was produced in the body.

This idea is now gaining more recognition, and a 1992 study in Finland, a country with one of the highest heart attack rates in the world, showed that high iron levels were a far better predictor of heart attacks than high cholesterol, high blood pressure, or diabetes. Men with a ferritin level of 200 or more in this study had the greatest risk of heart attacks. There have been other contradictory findings in this area, so more research is needed.

What is cholesterol?

Whenever you hear mention of the word "cholesterol," it is always negative. We are continually told to reduce our intake, lower the cholesterol we already have in our blood, or even take cholesterol-lowering drugs to bring the level down. Is cholesterol the "baddie" it is made out to be?

The answer is no. Basically, we need cholesterol: it is essential for life. From it our body makes all the sex hormones: estrogens, progesterone, and testosterone.

Confusion has arisen because there are two types of cholesterol. Dietary cholesterol is cholesterol contained in your food. Blood cholesterol is the type circulating in your body. It had been assumed that if you have too much cholesterol in your food it would automatically lead to too much cholesterol in your blood. This theory was tested and found wanting in 1975 by changing the diet of people with normal cholesterol levels. Two eggs, which are high in cholesterol, were given to twenty-five people every day for eight weeks. Another twenty-five people were given one egg every day for four weeks, then two eggs every day for the next four weeks. This made no difference to their blood cholesterol levels. It may be that the crucial factor is our bodies' ability to deal with the cholesterol, rather than just the quantity we eat.

Eggs, for instance, are high in cholesterol but low in saturated fats. Further research has shown that the amount of cholesterol in the blood seems to be linked to the amount of saturated fat we eat.

Cholesterol is manufactured in the liver and has a vital part to play in the structure of cells and the composition of certain hormones. Cholesterol is carried to the cells by LDL, low density lipoprotein, and then carried away to the liver to be excreted by HDL, high density lipoprotein. It is the levels of the LDL and HDL that are very important, far more important than the level of cholesterol. We are back to a question of balance. If the LDL ("bad") level is high and the HDL ("good") level is low, cholesterol will be deposited in the cells, but there will not be enough HDL to transport it away. The cholesterol can then be deposited in the artery walls by a process called atherosclerosis, which leads to narrowing and hardening of the arteries and then to heart disease.

It has also been found that if the cholesterol level from our food becomes too high, our liver will automatically manufacture less cholesterol. Again, given the chance, our bodies will keep us in balance and "know" exactly what should be happening, just like a thermostat on the heating system, turning the heat back on if the temperature in the house drops and turning it off if the house becomes too hot. For this to work efficiently, the heating system has to be well maintained and in good working order. The same principle applies to our bodies.

Ideally the amount of cholesterol in the blood should·be below 5.2. per quart (liter), LDL should be below 3.36, and HDL above 0.9. Some experts have suggested that a better measurement is the ratio of your cholesterol to HDL. A ratio of 3 to 1 is considered to be the best, 5 to 1 normal, and anything over that to be a high risk. Again, it is the balance that is important. As we will see, the kind of diet we eat is crucial to that balance.

Reducing the risk of a heart attack

1. **Reduce your iron intake**   We should really take iron only if we need it. Because iron is not eliminated from the body, we are just going to keep storing it. There is no benefit from having excess iron. Get your ferritin level checked, with a simple blood test. If the level is high, choose food supplements without iron and buy a non-fortified breakfast cereal. Also look carefully to see whether iron is hidden in any other foods you buy, such as bread or pasta.

2. **Keep an eye on your ferritin levels**   Ferritin levels in women still having periods should be between 12 and 40 micrograms per quart (liter) of blood. After the menopause they should be between 70 and 150. Checking involves a simple blood test which can be arranged with your doctor.

3. **Watch the saturated fats**   The usual recommendations for preventing heart disease, such as not smoking, exercising regularly, maintaining a sensible weight, and reducing saturated fats in your diet, still apply. If your diet is high in saturated fats and cholesterol and you have excess iron in your blood, you may be storing up trouble. You should reduce or even eliminate your intake of red meat, as this can mean double trouble because of its high cholesterol and high iron content.

4. **Keep an eye on your weight**   Weight gain is another important factor. The risk of heart disease seems to be

increased if you are carrying more weight around your waist and stomach than around your hips and thighs. After the menopause, however, fat distribution changes, and more can be deposited around the stomach area. If the ratio of your waist-to-hip measurement is more than 0.8, you can have a greater risk of heart disease, diabetes, osteoporosis, and arthritis, and you need to take preventive measures. To calculate your waist-to-hip ratio:

1. Measure your waist, finding where it is the narrowest.
2. Measure your hips at their widest point.
3. Divide your hip measurement by your waist measurement to calculate your ratio. For example:
   31in. (79cm.) waist ÷ 37in. (94cm.) hip = 0.84

How important is lifestyle?

Research has shown that heart disease is a degenerative disease linked to lifestyle factors. A degenerative disease means that the problems have been building up for a number of years. It is not just "one of those things." Dr. Weston Price, an American dentist, wrote a wide-ranging book entitled *Nutrition and Physical Degeneration*, published in 1970. His starting point was curiosity as to why dentists could not discover the cause of the dental decay and gum disease that are so common in the West. His researches took him all over the world, and he looked at different cultures as they changed their traditional diet to a more Western diet. He traced cultures and individuals over periods of ten years or more, watching the start and progress of many degenerative illnesses, including heart disease. He was one of the first people to realize that many modern illnesses are caused by our way of life.

We now know that heart disease can be prevented by adjusting what we eat and drink and our lifestyle. Unfortunately, many of the health messages we receive are negative—encouraging us to avoid this, that, or the next thing. This is important. But it's equally important to realize that the modern diet deprives us of essential nutrients that protect the body—and those nutrients need to come from the food we eat.

WHAT ABOUT THE "FRENCH PARADOX"?

The French consume at least the same amount of saturated fat as we do and possibly more, and yet their rate of heart disease is only 30 percent of ours. This fact puzzled the scientists, irritated the health information lobby, and cheered up the gourmets for years. Then we got the good news. It was probably the wine, especially red wine, that was protecting the French from heart problems. Then came the bad news. It seems that the protection is not from the alcohol in the wine but from the grapes the wine is made from. Grapes produce a substance called resveratrol, and in animal studies this has been shown to reduce blood fat and cholesterol levels. So you can forget the glass of wine and just have a bunch of grapes!

Onions and garlic, enjoyed by the French, also contain many organic sulfur compounds. The substances in garlic appear to work as a blood thinner in the same way as aspirin. The allicin in the garlic also seems to prevent cells from taking up cholesterol and reduces its production in the liver.

THE ESKIMOS

The Eskimos presented the scientists with another puzzle. They eat vast amounts of fat, and yet they have an extremely low rate of heart disease. The fat they eat comes from fish, which is known to be high in essential fatty acids, omega 3. These omega 3 oils have been found to lower cholesterol and triglycerides (fat stored in the body), decrease blood pressure, prevent blood clotting, and raise HDL (the cholesterol remover).

What can you do to help yourself?

First look at the risk factors listed below, and if any of them applies to you, take preventive measures to look after yourself:

- family history of heart disease,
- high blood lipids (cholesterol, triglycerides, LDLs),
- high blood pressure,
- smoking,
- obesity,
- lack of exercise,
- stress,
- earlobe crease.

Earlobe crease is at the bottom of the list because it is unusual. In fact it should go at the top. Having a diagonal crease in your earlobe has now been found to be a better predictor of heart problems than any of the other risk factors on the list. It was first linked to heart disease in 1973, and since then thirty studies have confirmed this finding.[8] Why is there this link? The earlobe has a rich supply of blood, so it is a good indicator of blood flow. If the supply of blood to the earlobe is restricted, over time a crease develops. So an earlobe crease can be a sign of restricted blood flow through the heart. It is interesting to note that in the West this link was first suspected in 1973, and yet traditional Oriental medicine has linked the ear to the heart for hundreds of years.

PREVENTIVE MEASURES

Do:

❑ **Include more oily fish, nuts, seeds, and oils in your diet** The essential fatty acids in these foods are important for the prevention of heart disease. The fish oils help to lower cholesterol, thin the blood, and lessen the risk of narrowing of the arteries. Walnuts have been shown to be helpful in preventing heart attacks, again due to the essential fatty acid content. A study of 26,500 Seventh Day Adventists, who do not drink or smoke, found that those who ate a handful of nuts at least five times a week had half the heart problems of those who rarely ate any nuts.[9] This underlines the crucial importance of diet in preventing heart disease.

❏ **Eat more fresh vegetables and fruit and also dried fruit** Fiber found in potatoes, carrots, apples, beans, and oats binds up the cholesterol and carries it out of the body. Vitamin C, found in fruit and vegetables, is important because low levels of vitamin C have been linked to increased levels of cholesterol.

❏ **Eat more soy** Soybeans have been found to help control cholesterol levels, so should be included in the diet in the form of tofu, soy milk, miso, tempeh, and tamari (wheat-free soy sauce made in the traditional way). Soybeans contain more protein than milk, without the saturated fat or cholesterol. They are the only beans considered to be a complete protein, because they contain all eight essential amino acids. Soy is also high in essential fatty acids. The role of soy in preventing and treating chronic disease has become so important that there is an annual four-day international conference devoted just to soy. The conference, hosted in Brussels in September 1996, with nearly eighty speakers from around the world, focused on the role of soy in reducing heart disease and cancer. And papers were presented on soy and hormones, the menopause, and osteoporosis.

❏ **Exercise regularly** Take brisk walks and get your heart beating faster than it usually does. Besides keeping the cardiovascular system in good condition, exercise also seems to help raise HDL (the ''good'' cholesterol) and lower LDL (the ''bad'' cholesterol).

❏ **Look at your vitamins** A very exciting confirmation of the link between good nutrition and heart disease came from a study published in *The Lancet* in March 1996. Scientists from Cambridge University and Papworth Hospital found that taking a daily dose of vitamin

E reduced the risk of having a heart attack by an astonishing 75 percent. An eighteen-month trial involved 2,000 patients with coronary arteriosclerosis (fatty deposits in the arteries). Half of the patients were given the vitamin E supplement with their regular medication and half took the placebo with their regular medication.[10]

The number of heart attacks in the group that took the vitamin E was a quarter of those taking the dummy pills. Those given the supplement appeared to be at no greater risk of having a heart attack than normal, healthy men and women of the same age with no heart problems.

According to Professor Morris Brown of Cambridge University, quoted in the *Journal of the Institute for Optimum Nutrition*:[11] "This is even more exciting than aspirin. Most people in our study were already taking aspirin. The average benefit from taking aspirin is in the order of 25 to 40 percent reduction. Vitamin E reduces the risk of heart attack by a massive 75 per cent."

Professor Brown then goes on to say that he would not suggest that people should stop taking aspirin. Why not? He just suggests that they take the vitamin E as well. He added, "It would be irresponsible for us to recommend it freely to those without heart disease." Is he actually suggesting you wait until you have narrowing of the arteries or a heart attack and then start the vitamin E?

With results like these on a large-scale double-blind controlled trial, doctors should be recommending what to eat and what to take to keep us well. But results like this and others before it get stuck in the academic literature without being put to any practical use. Several other previous studies, in fact, have indicated that vitamin E is important for heart health—low blood levels of this vitamin have been linked to heart attack risk.

- So increase your vitamin E intake from foods such as olives,. olive oil, avocado, and tuna, and take it in a supplement form.

❑ **Make sure your mineral levels are good**   It has been found that magnesium-rich foods seem to protect against coronary disease. A ten-year study of 2,000 men showed that those who had heart attacks had significantly less magnesium in their blood than those who did not. Also, analysis of three other trials has shown a significant reduction in deaths by treating heart disease patients with magnesium. Magnesium-rich foods are cereals such as wheat, oats, and rye.[12]

Don't:

• **Smoke**   The risk of heart attack is increased by 70 percent for smokers. Smoking thickens the blood, increasing the risk of clots, and also raises blood pressure.

Avoid:

• **Eating saturated fats and trans fatty acids**   Saturated fats are found in animal foods, including red meat, cheese, and milk. The trans fatty acids result from the hydrogenation of unsaturated fats into a solid form to make oils into margarine. Trans fatty acids have been linked to an increased rate of heart attacks. Before you buy that "low fat" or "polyunsaturated" spread, read the labels carefully. The manufacturing process not only destroys nutrients, it produces a food that cannot be properly metabolized by the body. In the United States, where the emphasis on marketing and buying "low fat" products has reached extreme proportions, it is believed that the switch to these hydrogenated oils, encouraged by health scares, may have done more harm than if people had just continued using old-fashioned butter.

FOR HEART PROTECTION

Take an all-around multivitamin and mineral for the menopause *plus* the following:

Linseed oil capsules—1,000mg. twice per day,
Vitamin C—1,000mg. twice per day,
Vitamin E—300ius per day,
Magnesium—150mg. per day.

Conclusion

Most specialists would agree that heart disease is over-whelmingly a lifestyle disease, caused by a combination of factors depending on each individual. There are plenty of ways that we can help ourselves reduce the risks. Eating sensibly, taking exercise, controlling stress, stopping smoking—these are commonsense approaches to decreasing the risk of heart disease, especially after the menopause.

As explained, the evidence that HRT protects against heart disease is far from conclusive—and even those experts who believe that supplemental estrogen may reduce the risks can't tell us *why*. It's quite disgraceful that women are being told that HRT can protect them when the state of real medical knowledge is so inexact and flimsy. In time, we may find that some women, perhaps those with particular high-risk factors, will get some protection from HRT and consider it worthwhile when balanced with the other risks of taking what is a very powerful drug. But it's hard to see how HRT could ever be recommended routinely to women as a protection against heart disease. None of us should be brainwashed into believing that HRT or any drug will ever be a substitute for a fundamentally "heart"-healthy lifestyle.

CHAPTER 10

How to control your weight and your mood

Some weight gain during the menopause is perfectly acceptable. As your ovaries reduce their production of hormones, your body fat acts as a manufacturing plant for estrogen. Those last 10 pounds (4.5kg.) you were trying to lose will serve you well. Fat produces estrogen all our lives. Being actually overweight is, of course, unhealthy. Ideally women should have 25 percent body fat in contrast to men's 15 percent. Women face a lot of pressure from the media and society in general to keep slim, and this, at the extreme, has resulted in a number of eating disorders like anorexia and bulimia. Many other women spend much of their lives yo-yo dieting, which in the end completely distorts their attitude to food. Yet statistics tell us that women are getting heavier on average, not lighter; in fact, obesity is a major health problem in the United States. Preparing for the menopause involves some hard thinking about your diet and nutrition. You may well find that changing your eating habits to a healthier pattern will, over time, bring about some of the elusive weight loss you have always longed for.

Why diets don't work

Dieting is a losing battle. As you reduce your food intake or skip meals, your body puts itself on "famine alert." It gets the impression that food is scarce, and therefore it slows down your metabolism to get the best use of the small amount of food. If you crash diet for a week and then go back to your normal pattern of eating, you will be consuming your normal diet with a slower metabolism so you will end up putting on weight far more easily. If you eat little and often, your body "knows" that food is plentiful. It doesn't need to store any excess in case there is a shortage, and it can keep your metabolism at a good level.

The conventional approach to weight loss has involved reducing calories. In scientific terms, a calorie is a unit of heat and the energy-producing property of food. The idea has been that if the calories going in are fewer than the calories being used up, the person will lose weight.

Food can be converted into fat or energy. We can either store what we eat or use it to do what we want with our lives. This happens through a number of chemical reactions, which are activated by enzymes, which are dependent in turn upon vitamins and minerals. Not all types of foods are easy to convert into energy.

You can eat more and weigh less. Some foods have a so-called "negative calorie" effect, and eating them actually helps you lose weight. Starchy foods, complex carbohydrates, boost your metabolism so you burn up calories more quickly and the body fat comes off. They do not add directly to body fat but they help you keep a good level of energy because they keep your blood sugar in balance. These foods include grains such as wheat, rice, oats, barley, and rye and foods made from these, such as bread and pasta. Potatoes are also classed as a complex carbohydrate.

Carbohydrates are broken down into a number of different sugars within the body. These sugars trigger the release of insulin, which then produces two hormones, noradrenaline and thyroid-stimulating hormone. Both of these help to stimulate the metabolism. This means that your food is burned more effectively and less is turned into fat. This is the negative-calorie effect. A portion of beef and a portion of rice may have the same number of calories, but they can have a radically different effect on your weight because of the body biochemistry involved.

By eating brown rice, whole-wheat bread, and pasta, as well as a good selection of fresh fruit and vegetables, you are also increasing the fiber content of your diet. In cultures where they have a diet high in fiber, they do not seem to have so many weight problems. Fiber helps to

- ❑ improve blood sugar balance,
- ❑ improve digestion and absorption,
- ❑ increase the excretion of fat in the stools,
- ❑ create a feeling of fullness, so you can feel satisfied more quickly without feeling the need to eat more.

So:

- ❑ eat more starchy foods;
- ❑ cut down on fatty and sugary foods—meat, poultry, all dairy products, margarine, cake, pie, ice cream, potato chips, sugary candies, and commercial salad dressing;
- ❑ don't count calories;
- ❑ avoid alcohol.

No-fat or low-fat diets are probably the most popular with women. But they are a bad idea, particularly for women going through the menopause. It's true that many Western diets contain too much fat. As much as 50 to 60 percent of our calorie intake is reckoned to come from fats. So by reducing our intake of saturated fats, it is possible to lose weight. However, there are certain unsaturated fats that are essential for our health; these are known as essential fatty acids (EFAs). It is unhealthy and counterproductive to go on a no-fat diet. Your body cannot make essential fats, so the only source is your diet. Totally fat-free diets have resulted in joint stiffness, skin problems, and vaginal dryness. These essential fats are a vital component of every human cell, and your body needs them to insulate your nerve cells, keep your skin and arteries supple, balance your hormones, and keep you warm. EFAs have been found to relieve benign breast disease. They increase metabolic rate and increase weight loss by stimulating fat burn-off.

These unsaturated essential fats are found in nuts (almonds, pecans, brazils, etc.), seeds (sesame, sunflower, pumpkin, etc.), oils (olive, sunflower, sesame), oily fish (tuna, mackerel), and vegetables.

It is the saturated fats that need to be kept to a minimum—the fats from animal foods such as dairy products (milk, cheese), eggs, poultry, and meats such as beef, lamb, and pork.

The best way to lose weight is to follow the recommendations in Chapter 5 and let the weight come off gradually. The more slowly weight comes off, the more likely it is to stay off. You need to find a way of eating that is a way of life. Not a diet that you follow for a while and then abandon for your old eating pattern but a way of eating that is enjoyable and nourishing and that allows your weight to remain stable.

Avoiding added sugar in the food you eat is crucial to losing weight. Sugar is just empty calories; it has no nutritional value, so it just adds on extra weight. It is obviously found in chocolate, cake, cookies, and candy. But it is hidden in many other foods, including main dishes and canned vegetables. It is an inexpensive bulking agent and tends to make us want to eat more of any food to which it has been added.

Sugar is in foods like ketchup, which contains only 8 percent less sugar than ice cream. Cream substitute for coffee has 65 percent sugar compared to 51 percent in a candy bar. It is not only hidden in our food but also in our drinks. A can of cola can contain eight teaspoons of sugar, and if we switch to a diet cola, we are just introducing unhealthful chemical sweeteners into our diet.

If you eat well, take proper exercise, and yet your weight does not shift, what do you do? First of all, check that you do not have a medical condition that is causing the weight gain, such as an underactive thyroid. Symptoms of an underactive thyroid (hypothyroidism) include difficulty in losing weight, depression, headaches, lack of energy, dry skin, menstrual problems, and constipation. A blood test is usually performed to assess your thyroid function, although it has been found that it is not very accurate in detecting mild forms of underactivity. Before the advent of this test, the most popular way of testing thyroid function was by measuring the basal body temperature, and that is still a valid test today.

Your body temperature is a good guide to the state of your metabolism. To test your thyroid function you need to measure your basal body temperature, which is your temperature at rest. First get a thermometer. There are some good electronic ones on the market which take only a minute to register the temperature and bleep when they have done it.

❏ Put the thermometer by your bed before you go to sleep.
❏ When you wake in the morning, put the thermometer in your armpit and leave it until it bleeps. Your temperature needs to be taken with you lying as still as possible. Do not get out of bed or have a drink before you take your temperature.
❏ Record your temperature in the same way over three mornings. It needs to be taken at the same time each morning.
❏ If you are still having periods, you need to do this test on the second, third, and fourth day of your cycle. Your body temperature rises after ovulation, so it would not give a clear picture of what is happening to take your temperature later in the cycle. Your basal body temperature should read between 97.6 and 98.2°F (36.4 and 36.7°C).

If the temperature is low, it would be advisable to speak to your doctor about possible problems with your thyroid.

Weight gain also often follows a hysterectomy. I have seen women who have put on 28 pounds (12.7kg.) or more after this operation. This level of weight gain is also often linked to taking HRT, so make sure you have eliminated all possible causes for the weight gain.

Once you have checked these possibilities, there are a number of other ways to try to lose weight. First try a food-combining regime based on avoiding eating proteins and starches together at the same meal. The theory is that both protein and starches need different enzymes to be digested, so there will be a ''fight'' as both cannot be digested effectively at the same time. This theory does not seem to have been proven scientifically, and yet people get very good results by trying it. This ''fight'' can cause bloating and weight gain because the undigested food is being stored and not properly assimilated. Women who have lost weight using food combining often choose to eat this way permanently, as they feel it gives them more energy and fewer digestive troubles. The easiest way to understand this method of eating is to follow a few simple rules:

1. Don't mix starchy food with proteins.
2. Eat fruit by itself.
3. Don't have milk with either starch or protein.

Food allergies

The term ''food allergy'' has been used to describe an adverse reaction to a particular food. It is thought that all allergies involve an immune-system response. For some people this response is almost immediate. Common foods that are linked to this type of allergy are shellfish, strawberries, and, even more severe, peanuts. The person may develop a rash, get diarrhea or constipation, or, in extreme cases, go into severe shock (anaphylaxis).

Masked food allergies, however, have a much more delayed response, and the effects can be quite deceptive but may cause a number of symptoms such as weight gain, bloating, water retention, stomach disorders, aching joints, fatigue, stuffy nose, skin problems, asthma, hyperactivity, and migraine headaches. If you are allergic to a particular food, it is likely that you will crave it and eat it frequently. The food becomes mildly addictive. You may find it hard to believe you are reacting to it.

How can you track down a food allergy? There are two ways to do this: have a blood test or follow a hypoallergenic diet.

BLOOD TEST

A sample of your blood is used to test whether your immune system is reacting in the presence of certain foods. There are a number of ways this immune response is measured, and these are described in Chapter 12, "Tests at the Menopause" (see page 222). Once you know which foods you react to, these can be removed from your diet.

HYPOALLERGENIC DIET

This is a self-help system designed to track down food allergies. You take out those foods and drinks that are most likely to be indicated in food allergy and follow the hypoallergenic diet for about two weeks. The diet is reproduced here by kind permission of the Society for the Promotion of Nutritional Therapy.

You may eat:

All fresh vegetables Includes raw vegetables and salads, lightly steamed or stewed vegetables, soups made with fresh vegetables, potatoes (without butter). Frozen vegetables. Do not use canned vegetables except for pulses.

All fresh fruits and pure fruit juices Canned fruit is occasionally allowed if it contains fruit juice with no sugar, rather than syrup.

All fresh or frozen fish Oily fish like mackerel, herrings, and sardines are especially recommended. Canned fish is acceptable if in pure oil, brine, or spring water.

All fresh or roasted nuts and seeds (unsalted) Includes almonds, brazils, walnuts, cashews, hazelnuts, and pecans. Sesame seeds and linseeds need to be ground up first, otherwise they just pass straight through you. Other seeds to include are sunflower seeds, pumpkin seeds, pine kernels. Tahini (sesame seed paste) and other nut butters are fine as long as they are sugar- and additive-free.

All pulses   Includes lentils, chickpeas, kidney beans, lima beans, butter beans, haricot beans, aduki beans. You can cook these yourself or buy canned. If you are cooking kidney beans and chickpeas, remember that they need to be soaked overnight. The soaking water should then be discarded and the beans cooked very thoroughly in fresh water. Check that canned beans do not contain sugar or anything else except salted water.

All soy products   Includes tofu, soy milk, miso. Use tamari instead of soy sauce for flavoring, as it is wheat-free but soy sauce is not; sometimes soy sauce contains MSG (monosodium glutamate), which should be avoided.

All cold-pressed (unrefined) oils   Includes sesame, sunflower, extra-virgin olive oil. The supermarket oils (except extra-virgin olive oil) often contain anti-foaming agents and other chemicals added in the processing to extract more oil and should be avoided.

Non-gluten grains   Includes brown rice, millet, and buckwheat, as well as flours and flakes made from these grains. Since grains are very small, they can absorb more pesticide, so try to buy organically grown ones if available. Use arrowroot or corn-starch as thickeners.

Pure herbal or fruit teas   Includes peppermint, camomile, rosehip, etc.

Natural sweeteners   Honey (in small amounts), maple syrup, rice syrup, date syrup.

You may not eat:

Dairy products   Butter, cheese, milk, yogurt, or anything containing dairy products, lactose or whey, including sheep's and goats' milk products.

Gluten grains   Wheat, oats, and any others except those on the "allowed" list. These grains can be in bread, pastry, sauces and gravies, pasta, batter, cake, or cookies.

Stock cubes/powders or gravy/sauce mixes These should be avoided, as they can contain disguised wheat (in the form of hydrolyzed vegetable protein) or yeast. Use miso paste dissolved in hot water and add to the dish, but do not boil once the miso is added.

Animal products Red meat, poultry, eggs.

Stimulants Sugar, tea, coffee, alcohol, beer, wine. Do not eat candy or chocolate.

Artificial additives Colorings, preservatives, "instant" or convenience foods, etc.

Yeast Yeast extracts, fermented foods, sauces or drinks (except miso or tamari).

This is a hypoallergenic diet. Unlike some diets, it places no restriction on the quantity of food you can eat, only on the types. Get organized, so that you are well stocked with foods you are allowed and don't feel deprived. Try to plan to adopt this diet when you have some degree of control over your meals and not too many social events coming up. You may still get good results even if you can follow it for only a week.

For the first few days you may feel worse, as your body begins to eliminate toxins and waste products. You may also get withdrawal symptoms from certain stimulants such as tea and coffee. You may feel as if you are coming down with the flu, feel headachy, or get diarrhea or aches and pains. But persevere and I can assure you there is light at the end of the tunnel. Most women say they get a feeling of having so much more energy after they have completed the diet.

HOW TO ADD FOODS BACK IN

Once you've had a blood test and eliminated the reactive foods or you have done the hypo-allergenic diet, what then?

This is the important step, especially if you have followed the hypo-allergenic diet, because you can now find out what is causing your weight gain and any other related symptoms. Take one type of food only, such as wheat, and add it back in on one day only. Then stop the wheat and monitor yourself for two or three days. Note how you are feeling: do you feel bloated, tired? Do you have joint pains? Or is there no difference? If at the end of the three days you do not feel any different, add in another type of food, such as dairy foods, for one day. If you had a reaction after adding in the wheat, take it out and wait for yourself to stabilize again before adding in the next food. Keep a note of your reaction. This is called food challenging and is a very effective way to track down your allergies.

If you are not sure of your reaction to a particular food, you can double-check by taking your pulse. It has been found that food allergy can cause an increase in pulse rate.

Pulse test

1. Count your pulse while sitting after resting for a few minutes. You can find your pulse on the thumb side of your wrist. Count how many pulses in thirty seconds and double your answer.
2. Add in the food that you are challenging, then take your pulse ten minutes later. It is also valuable to take it again after thirty minutes and then after one hour. If you are allergic to a particular substance, your pulse rate can increase by ten points or more.

Extra help for weight loss

A number of chemical reactions are involved in turning glucose into energy instead of fat. These are controlled by enzymes, which are themselves dependent on certain vitamins and minerals in the body. If these are deficient, you will lack energy and feel low. So while it is important to identify any allergies and to eat well, you can also help yourself by making sure that you are taking a good balance of vitamins and minerals. While you are restricting your food to check on the allergies, it can be a good idea to take some supplements to ensure that you have a good balance of nutrients.

The B vitamins are important, especially vitamins B3 and B6, and the minerals zinc and chromium. They help to supply fuel to cells ready for burning to give you energy. Vitamin B6 is especially important because it is needed for the production of pancreatic enzymes which help effective digestion. Together with zinc, B6 is needed to make the enzyme that digests food.

Zinc is an important mineral in appetite control, and a deficiency of zinc can cause a loss of taste and smell so that we crave and seek stronger-tasting foods. Chromium is needed for the metabolism of sugar. Without it insulin is less effective in controlling blood sugar levels. Chromium also helps to control levels of fat and cholesterol in the blood.

Vitamin C can play a role in weight control, too. It helps to lower cholesterol and is involved in the conversion of glucose to energy in the cells.

Co-enzyme Q10 is important for energy production. It's found in all the tissues and organs of our bodies, but as we get older we may become deficient. Any deficiency of co-enzyme Q10 results in a reduction of energy and a slowing down of the life-giving process. It has been used to help heart problems, high blood pressure, gum disease, and immune deficiencies.[1] A study showed that people on a low-fat diet doubled their weight loss when supplemented with Q10 compared to those who did not have the extra Q10.[2]

Garcinia cambogia, a small tropical fruit form Central Asia, where the rind is used in Thai and Indian cooking, can also help with weight loss. The garcinia contains HCA (hydroxy-citric acid) which can enable carbohydrates to be turned into usable energy instead of being deposited as fat. The HCA in this fruit seems to curb appetite, reduce food intake, and inhibit the formation of fat and cholesterol; though this has yet to be proven scientifically. *Garcinia cambogia* is marketed under the brands Citrimax and Rainbow Light.

Eating, of course, is not a purely mechanistic biochemical process. Food is and should be enjoyable, appealing to our senses. Constant dieting can distort our emotional relationship with food. Not eating the right food at the right time can also affect our moods and emotions, sabotaging our efforts to establish a healthy eating pattern that will result in weight loss.

The psychology of food

Food and our mood go together. When we are depressed, we cheer ourselves up with a chocolate bar. There are substances in chocolate that do indeed impart the "feel good" factor—the same chemical buzz that we get when we are in love. In the September 1996 edition of *Nature*, researchers showed that the chemicals in chocolate targeted the same brain receptors as marijuana, suggesting that both chocolate and marijuana may share a similar chemistry. Chocolate's effect was definitely milder than marijuana's, but it may explain why chocolate is eaten at times of stress or depression.

Scientists have now found that foods can trigger all kinds of important changes in our brain chemistry. What we eat and drink can determine whether we feel happy or depressed. These powerful brain chemicals can also affect our appetite and our ability to control it. Many of us eat more when we are feeling sad, lonely, and depressed. We eat for comfort and to ward off boredom. Becoming aware of what controls your appetite and eating patterns is crucial when it comes to losing weight and establishing a healthy diet.

Brain chemicals are neurotransmitters which transmit signals to neurones (brain cells). Some of these brain chemicals can control our appetite. They either make us eat more or make us eat less.

BRAIN CHEMICALS

These brain chemicals increase our intake of food:

• endorphins,
• norepinephrine (noradrenaline),
• neuropeptide Y.

These decrease our intake of food:

- cholecystokinin (CCK),
- serotonin,
- corticotropin-releasing factor.

So we are back to the idea of balance again. We need to feel hungry to keep ourselves alive, and yet we also need to feel satisfied to know when to stop eating.

How do these brain chemicals make us feel?

Serotonin makes us feel calm and sleepy and can lift depression. Norepinephrine (noradrenaline) makes us feel alert and energetic. Endorphins can give us a "natural buzz," a sense of euphoria.

Complex carbohydrates such as pasta, potatoes, and bread increase the levels of serotonin which control our appetite and make us feel good. A high-carbohydrate meal causes a larger proportion of tryptophan, an amino acid, to get to the brain to stimulate the production of serotonin. Carbohydrates help the body to release insulin, and this increases the uptake of the other amino acids, leaving the tryptophan to dominate.

On the other hand, when we eat a protein meal or snack, a number of amino acids including tryptophan are competing to get into the brain, and therefore the tryptophan cannot dominate.

So complex carbohydrates make us feel happier and more relaxed and control our appetite for the next meal. Eating little and often and keeping our blood sugar in balance enables us to control our moods and also our appetites without feeling deprived or hungry.

Protein contains an amino acid called tyrosine which manufactures the neurotransmitters norepinephrine (noradrenaline) and dopamine, which helps to focus our mind and keep us alert.

Understanding the different biochemical reactions of food on our mood enables us to use it to our advantage.

Having a carbohydrate breakfast has a positive mood-enhancing effect. But since a mainly carbohydrate meal can make us feel relaxed and sleepy, it may be better to have a predominantly protein meal for lunch so that we can feel alert and focused for the afternoon. The body naturally has a "post-lunch dip" in the afternoon. So if you have a carbohydrate meal at lunch you may find that it is difficult to keep your eyes open.

It is important to eat breakfast, but if you find that this makes you feel hungry all day, you should eat a protein breakfast. If you crave candy and chocolates mid afternoon, you need to eat carbohydrates for lunch and also as an afternoon snack. If you feel tired after lunch, eat a protein lunch, and if you are turning to alcohol to help you relax in the evening, have a mainly carbohydrate evening meal. We are all different. Look at your own daily pattern and work out what different kinds of food are appropriate, and at which times, for you.

There are other ways of controlling your appetite. The chemical cholecystokinin (CCK) is released as food enters the stomach. It tells the digestion to slow down and then gives the message to the brain that you are "full," and your appetite naturally decreases. This message takes time, therefore you need to eat more slowly so that your body knows when you have had enough.

Interestingly, the neurotransmitter neuropeptide Y is increased in those who exercise. This brain chemical increases our appetite but makes us want to eat complex carbohydrates, which release serotonin, which makes us feel good and keeps our appetite under control.

Along with brain chemicals, psychological factors play a strong part in food urges. Food is often given as a reward to children or when they are sad or crying. Even the memory of pleasant experiences can cause food cravings.

WHAT CAN YOU DO ABOUT FOOD CRAVINGS?

1. **Know your triggers** Become aware of when you crave certain foods. If you know that certain situations

make you feel the need for certain foods, either avoid the situations if possible or else prepare yourself by taking something else to eat that may satisfy that need.

2. **Are your emotions a trigger?**   Are you eating differently when you feel sad, lonely, or bored? Look at what else you could substitute instead of food. Perhaps do some volunteer work to shift the emphasis away from yourself. This can help with any feelings of self-pity. Find a new hobby or join an evening class—learn to scuba dive! Bring some excitement into your life.

3. **Habit eating**   It is very easy to get into habits such as eating while driving or eating while watching TV. These can become so ingrained that you can end up always eating while watching TV. Have a look at what has become automatic. A patient came to see me who had got into the habit of coming home from work and automatically going to the fridge. This action had almost become unconscious. Awareness of what you are doing and when is the key. Stop, think, and ask yourself, ''Do I really need to eat this now? Will I be happy with the way I feel after I have eaten it?''

4. **Exercise**   Exercise releases chemicals called endorphins which make us feel good. Going for a brisk walk or a swim when you feel cravings can even ward off the urge to binge.

5. **Go for complex carbohydrates**   Complex carbohydrates—starchy foods such as rice, potatoes, millet, wheat, rye, oats, and barley—keep the blood sugar in balance so that your body automatically stops craving a ''quick fix.'' Because complex carbohydrates burn slowly, they help us to feel satisfied with less food and also give us a good level of energy. It's the difference between burning coal and newspaper on a fire. The complex carbohydrates are the coal. They slowly build up heat and keep up a good level of warmth over a long period of time. The newspaper, however, gives a quick burst of heat, and then you have to fuel the fire again. You will be amazed that you can eat filling and satisfying food, feel good, and still lose weight.

6. **Distract yourself**   What if you wait for the craving to subside? Yes, they do go, even if you don't satisfy them. Do something else, read, or make a phone call, and see what you feel like after that.

7. **Eat little and often**   Do not go more than three hours without food. Your blood sugar level will drop, and then your body will automatically crave something sweet as a "quick fix." If you leave a large gap between meals, you can actually end up eating far more. Long gaps increase the chemical neuropeptide Y in the brain, which actually increases your hunger. Long gaps between meals can also put your body into the famine mode and slow your metabolism down so you can end up putting on more weight. This is why constant dieting makes you fat.

8. **Don't deny yourself**   If you say to yourself you are never going to eat chocolate again, you will almost certainly fail. Be realistic. We are all going to have foods that we are really better off without. If the main foundation of your nutrition is good, relax, go away on vacation, and enjoy yourself. If you are out with a friend for a treat, don't feel excluded if you want to have an ice cream with them. Buy the best quality you can get of that ice cream, and really become aware of the taste when you eat it. If you keep denying yourself, the craving can just explode, so that you end up eating far more than before. It becomes an obsession. If you eat little and often, with good amounts of complex carbohydrates, you will find the cravings will go automatically, without your having to use much willpower.

Jane came to see me knowing that during the week before each period she would sit and eat a box of chocolates every afternoon: she just couldn't stop herself. I explained to her about the blood sugar swings and cravings and she agreed to eat little and often during her next cycle, with more emphasis on complex carbohydrates. She said to me, "This isn't going to work." I replied, "What have you got to lose by trying it? Only the cravings." I saw her after her next period and she was just amazed. She was amazed not only that the cravings had gone but also at the way they had gone. It wasn't a case of willpower—''I will not eat chocolate''—but that her body didn't need the chocolate, so it didn't ask her for it. She had gone through the whole month without thinking about chocolate. She had even been out for dinner, was offered an after-dinner mint, and felt she could just take it or leave it. And she left it.

CHAPTER 11

The benefits of exercise and sex at the menopause

It's hard to exaggerate the benefits of regular exercise, it really is. And the older you get, the more important exercise is for your health. It has a direct impact on the way you feel and look as well as on your bone strength, your heart function, and your hormones. Regular exercise appears to be linked to a lower risk of breast cancer and a higher tolerance of stress, and it is absolutely vital for any woman who wants to keep a youthful figure, good skin, and a general zest for life.

Your emotions

Exercise releases brain chemicals called endorphins, which help us to feel happier, more alert, and calmer. Just exercise on its own has been shown to have a dramatic positive effect on people suffering from depression, stress, anxiety, and insomnia, and it is now often recommended as part of the treatment for these problems.

Your bone health

Weight bearing and weight training help maintain bone density through the menopause and prevent osteoporosis. Weight-bearing exercises include brisk walking, running, tennis, badminton, stair climbing, and aerobics—any activity that puts stress on your bones. Women who have allowed themselves to become inactive are at risk of fractures later on in life. It is definitely a case of "use it or lose it." Our bodily functions are very logical. Astronauts lose bone density in the weightlessness of space where there is no pressure on their bones. The same principle applies to the rest of us. If we make the demands on our body to provide us with good strong bones, bone density will be maintained or increased. When the bones are put under stress and their strength is in demand, the body will draw osteoblasts (bone builders) to those areas that need building up. If we become inactive and make no demands on our bones, we are compromising our bone health.

The impact of exercise on bone has been dramatically illustrated by research that examined the difference in bone density between the two arms of professional tennis players. The bones of the racket-holding arm, which does most of the work, can be over a third denser than those in the other one.[1] Several studies have shown that weight-bearing exercise helps women maintain or increase their bone density through and beyond the menopause.[2] At the same time we have to be careful about putting too much strain on our joints. A recent study reported in the British *Journal of Arthritis and Rheumatism* compared former first-class athletes with a group of ordinary women with an average age of fifty-two. The researchers, from St. Thomas's Hospital, London, were looking at the difference in osteoporosis between the two groups and the rate of osteoarthritis (wear and tear on the joints). The former athletes had 15 percent stronger bones than the other women but a greater risk of osteoarthritis. Clearly the answer is to find forms of exercise that put demands on the bones but avoid too much pressure on joints. The recommendation of the St. Thomas's team was that we should have an hour's weight-bearing exercise a week, or two hours of walking spread out over a week if we don't want to go to the gym. The researchers felt there were benefits from short bursts of activity, such as running for ten minutes, as long as it was done every day.

Because our lifestyles have changed, we need to make an effort to get enough of the right kind of exercise. In my mother's generation, exercise came naturally as part of the everyday routine. Both my father and mother would walk a few miles to work and back each day. After my sister and I were born, my mother would walk to get fresh vegetables and groceries each day and carry them back. Washing was done weekly by hand and involved a lot of scrubbing and wringing out of clothes (strengthening the back and the wrists). Every job required more effort and was physically demanding. What do I do? I put the family's clothes in the washing machine, turn it on, and then take the clothes out. I drive the car to the stores once a week to pick up the shopping. In order for me to keep active, exercise needs to be a conscious part of my life. I deliberately choose to walk up stairs instead of taking the elevator, I walk up escalators, I run up the stairs at home. I park the car farther away from the stores and have to walk (except when doing the main shopping for the week). None of us would want to go back to the days when the household jobs took so much more hard physical effort, but we have to find some way of making up for the lack of everyday exercise in our lives.

Exercise isn't important just for our bone health. It also helps keep our reflexes sharp and improves our coordination. Many fractures happen because someone falls or misses a step. If you keep yourself flexible and have good reflexes and coordination, you may save yourself from falling in the first place. As we get older, our range of movement becomes limited unless we make the effort through exercise to maintain it. Exercise also helps build up our muscles—and strong muscles act as the first line of defense when we have an accident, shielding our bones from the impact.

Your appetite

Besides releasing the feel-good endorphins, exercise stimulates other brain chemicals. Corticotropin releasing factor (CRF), for example, suppresses appetite, so that after exercise you simply don't want to stuff yourself with food even though you have used up plenty of calories. Even after this effect wears off, the kind of food your body demands is very different. Another brain chemical released by regular exercise is neuropeptide. This is the neurotransmitter that increases our need for carbohydrates—it "tells" our body what kind of fuel it needs. Carbohydrates are the body's prime source of energy. Fat and, to a lesser degree, protein, give us energy, too. But the main source should be carbohydrates, the starchy foods, like rice, potatoes, wheat, rye, and oats, which should ideally make up about half our calorie intake. So when we exercise, which uses up energy, our bodies release brain chemicals that make us eat more of the foods that give us more energy. It's a very clever system which demonstrates yet again how our bodies, given the chance, will find the right balance.

Your love life

When we are full of energy and vitality, we are much more interested in sex. You may feel you are just too tired to have sex. But by actually doing exercises that require effort and energy in the first place, you will end up feeling much more energized. You know how your interest in sex can perk up when you are on vacation? There are no pressures, you are more relaxed, and you also have more energy. Why wait for this to happen perhaps once a year? Get yourself fit and active, and enjoy making love.

Exercises like swimming and cycling which promote the blood supply to the vaginal area can help with vaginal dryness. Special exercises developed by Dr. Arnold Kegel in the 1940s can also make sex more enjoyable by increasing the strength of your vaginal sensations. They counteract vaginal dryness because they stimulate the blood supply. And they strengthen the muscles in the pelvic area which helps with stress incontinence ("leaking" small amounts of urine when you laugh or sneeze).

These are some of the simplest exercises to do. First of all try stopping your urine flow in midstream by finding and using the relevant vaginal muscles. Once you have located these muscles, you can exercise them by just contracting them whenever you think of doing it. Draw the muscles up for a count of five and then relax. Repeat this about ten times. You can also use these muscles while actually having intercourse: squeeze your partner's penis just by contracting them.

I found that these exercises really helped me. After the birth of my third child, who was a fairly large 9 lbs. 9 oz. (4.3kg.), I suspected a vaginal prolapse, which then seemed to rectify itself. A couple of years later I had the dragging feeling again, and consulted my doctor. He confirmed that I had a slight prolapse, and told me to come back for treatment when it had gotten worse. I found this rather unhelpful. My objective was not to let it get any worse, in case it reached the point where I might have to have a hysterectomy. So, deciding to practice what I preach, I looked for some alternatives. I went to see an acupuncturist, took herbs and food supplements, and did the Kegel exercises. Ten years later I still feel fine. It could be argued that perhaps the herbs on their own would have worked, or just the acupuncture, and that it was nothing to do with the exercises. Perhaps. Whether it was one of those or a combination of all three, it worked.

There are other exercises that help keep the circulation going and enhance your sex life.

THE PELVIC TILT

Lie on your back with your knees bent and feet flat on the floor. Slowly tilt and curl your pelvis. Hold for twenty seconds and then let go. Continue for five minutes.

THE BOW

Standing with your hands on your hips, breathe deeply and then bend your knees. Suck in your stomach and arch your back. Hold for twenty seconds and then let go. Repeat for five minutes.

Your heart

Exercise increases the circulation and also seems to lower LDL (the "bad" cholesterol) and increase HDL (the "good" cholesterol). The improvement in circulation is especially good for varicose veins. Exercise will allow the blood to keep circulating freely instead of becoming obstructed. "Tired" or "heavy" legs respond well to regular walking or jogging. Regular exercise can help to reduce blood pressure, one of the main risk factors for heart disease.

Your weight

Exercise allows us to burn fat more efficiently. It boosts our metabolism, so that we burn off calories at a faster rate even after we've stopped exercising. Exercise is particularly important if you are on a diet, since it keeps your metabolism going. Otherwise your metabolism can slow down when you reduce the amount of food you eat. How many calories do you burn off doing everyday activities? This is how many you can use up in twenty minutes:

Activity	Calories burned
Ironing	20
Doing housework	60
Mowing the lawn	60
Digging the garden	100
Walking upstairs	120
Running upstairs	200

Your general health

Exercise can have a powerful all-around effect on your health. Apart from the feelings of well-being, there are other physical benefits. Regular exercise has been shown to help with insomnia. Moderate exercise performed at a time of day other than just before bed has helped improve sleep quality.

Regular activity helps to keep our bowels working efficiently, which means we are eliminating waste products the body doesn't need. Exercise, in fact, is a prime treatment for constipation. Along with this, it improves the function of the immune system, the lymph system, and the ability of the body to keep our blood sugar in balance.

Your hormones

Exercise helps to keep your adrenal glands healthy. This is crucially important at the menopause, because the adrenals convert androstenadione into estrone, which is the main source of estrogen after the menopause. Your adrenals perch on top of your kidneys and consist of two parts, the medulla and cortex. The medulla secretes the stress hormones adrenaline and noradrenaline (norepinephrine), and the cortex produces three kinds of hormones including the sex hormones. Adrenaline and noradrenaline should be brought into play only when you are in a "fight or flight" situation. At a time of danger, you are geared up either to run or to defend yourself. To do this, your body goes through a number of changes. The response is immediate and dramatic. Your liver releases stored sugar into your bloodstream in case you need instant energy. Blood is taken away from the skin and moved into muscles and internal organs. Your heart speeds up and arteries tighten to raise your blood pressure to move the blood to where it is needed the most. Your digestion shuts down because you don't need to think about digesting a sandwich now: your energy is needed elsewhere. At the same time, your blood thickens, ready to clot in case you are injured.

All this happens very fast and should last for only a short space of time, enough to get you out of danger. The danger is then over, and you can recuperate. But our modern life-styles create different kinds of stresses. What happens if you are stuck in a traffic jam, late for an appointment, getting more and more stressed, and eating your lunch at the same time? All the stress responses will kick into play just the same. The difference is that in the "fight or flight" situation, you would have taken some action, run, or fought. In the traffic jam, you just sit there and seethe. Also, it is not going to be short-lived because you could be in that traffic jam for thirty minutes. Your digestion has shut down and you are trying to eat. The clotting time of your blood is shorter, so what is that going to do to your risk of heart attacks and strokes?

People nowadays often live their lives in a state of stress. Constant demands are made on the adrenal glands, to the point where they can become exhausted. It's not just the traffic jam. It's the pressure of work, the pressure of family, money worries. Every day there are numerous instances in which the body is put on what is a biochemical "red alert." The health of your adrenal glands is important at any stage of your life, but especially so at the menopause. As your ovaries slow down their production of sex hormones, your adrenal glands will take over that process, producing not only estrone, a form of estrogen, but also androgens (male hormones), which are the ones that give you drive and zest. Exercise gives your body the proper physical outlet for all that stress, enabling your hormone systems to get back in balance. If the body has no physical outlet for all this "inactive" stress, you suffer symptoms like backache, shoulder pain, tension headaches, digestive problems, ulcers, and high blood pressure.

Can you have too much exercise?

The answer is yes. Too much exercise can cause a change in the body–fat ratio and stop periods (amenorrhea). Very young gymnasts and athletes have found that over-exercising has prevented their periods from even beginning. This type of athletic amenorrhea results from hormonal imbalance and carries the risk of reduced bone mineral density later on in life. At the menopause we need some body fat, so that, as our ovaries shut down, estrogen can be produced from our fat cells. Heavy exercise, running, or going to the gym every day, for instance, or training for a particular event, can put the body under more stress than the exercise is relieving. More nutritional demands will be made, and excessive sweating can cause the loss of vital minerals such as zinc, potassium, sodium, etc. Most of us, of course, come nowhere near to over-exercising. But some women become "hooked" on it—often women who have had eating problems when they were younger. Again we come back to the idea of balance and moderation.

How to design your own exercise program

Since regular exercise is more beneficial than "big bursts" you need to find something that you enjoy and that motivates you enough for you to want to do it regularly. Brisk walking is very beneficial and can be fitted in at any time. It does not require special equipment or clothing and is inexpensive. It is a good weight-bearing exercise, so can help to protect the bones. It can also free the mind, so that your imagination can just "wander off," while you are walking. If you have not exercised for years, walking is a good way to start getting fit. If you have not picked up a tennis racket since you were at school, *don't* rush out onto the tennis court and start playing furiously. That is a sure-fire recipe for a bad muscle injury.

We are all individuals, so we have to find an exercise routine that fits in with our families, our lifestyle, and our finances. Some women will prefer to exercise on their own; others need the motivation of a group or a friend to keep them going. Use whatever you need to keep active and fit.

If you have not been exercising regularly, take things slowly at first and build up gradually. Your pulse rate is a good indicator of how fit you are and can help you to know if you are overdoing it when exercising. The more unfit you are, the faster your pulse is, because the heart has to work harder to pump blood around your body. Find the pulse in your wrist by placing three fingertips on the bone running down from your thumb. Move your fingers inward until you feel the beat of your pulse. Count the number of beats in thirty seconds and then double your answer to get your pulse per minute. Your maximum pulse rate is 220 minus your age. So if you are forty-five, your maximum pulse rate will be $220 - 45 = 175$. When you are exercising check your pulse rate after about three to four minutes. If you are unfit, you should aim for a pulse rate of 60 percent of your maximum; if you are fit, this can rise to 80 per cent.

To check if you are exercising at the right level, look at the table below:

Age	Target rate during exercise 60 percent if unfit	Target rate during exercise 80 percent if fit
40	108	144
45	105	140
50	99	132
55	96	128

WHAT KIND OF EXERCISE?

You need weight-building exercise for the bones, aerobic exercise for your heart and circulation, and some kind of stretching exercise to keep you flexible and poised. My time is very limited, so I have chosen a variety of exercises to give me all-around benefits. Some I can do at home and some I need to plan. I mix walking, running up the stairs, yoga, exercises from a video, and a visit to my local health club, which has a gym. That way I get all the different kinds of exercise my body needs.

Many years ago I was taught a series of yoga movements called the Sun Salutation, and they have stayed with me ever since. The Sun Salutation is taught as an exercise to start the day, but you can do it at other times. I like it because there is a definite start and finish and also because of the variety of movements it offers in one simple sequence. The benefits are many, including posture, deep breathing, spine stretching, improved flexibility, increased circulation, and relaxation. Strictly speaking the Sun Salutation sequence is those movements numbered 1–4 and back again, as illustrated opposite, but I do the sequence twice to exercise both sides of the body (illustrations 1–12). Depending on the time available, you can repeat it any number of times.

Swimming is not weight-bearing. But if you enjoy it, you should do it to increase stamina, improve your cardiovascular health, and get a good stretch. There may be an aqua aerobics class at your local pool. That is an excellent way to get cardiovascular exercise and tone your muscles without putting pressure on your joints. And if you are on the plump side, you will be more adept at it than thinner women, whose lack of body fat makes it harder for them to float.

As with food, you should try to introduce variety so that your body gets all the different kinds of exercise it needs. Start with thirty minutes of exercise once a week and gradually build up to one hour, three times per week, of various kinds of exercise. Whatever you do, be sure to first warm up properly by doing some stretching exercises. This reduces the risk of injury to your muscles and joints. If you join an exercise class, make sure the instructor is properly trained and that he or she teaches you to do the exercises in the right way. It is easy to damage your back by pulling on the wrong muscles.

Because of limited time and wanting to fit in exercise whenever I can, I have used an exercise video at home. There are some excellent exercise videos on the market, but also be aware that some should be treated with caution. I have found the videos by Katy Smith to be particularly useful. These have a number of sections, and I find that if I have only fifteen minutes to spare I can choose a complete section to follow.

Exercises for your breasts

There are no muscles in the breasts. Toning the pectoral muscles in your chest, however, can help your breasts to

Sun Salutation

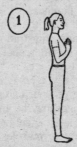

1

Stand up straight, shoulders back, feet together, arms hanging loosely at your sides. Breathe deeply and exhale as you bring your hands together in front of you.

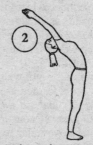

2

Inhale and stretch your arms out over your head. Roll your hips forward and arch back from the waist, pushing your head back.

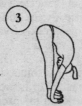

3

Exhale and slowly bend forward from the waist, placing your hands flat on the ground on either side of your feet, so that your fingers and toes form a straight line.

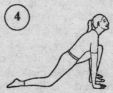

4

Inhale and, keeping your hands and feet in the same position, stretch your right leg back and drop your right knee to the ground.

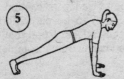

5

Holding your breath, take your left leg back. Straighten both legs and hold your body in a straight diagonal.

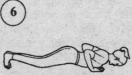

6

Exhale, bend your knees, and place your knees, chest, and forehead on the ground, raising your buttocks. Keep your elbows tucked in close to your body.

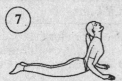

7

Inhale, slide your hips forward, point your toes back, and arch your head and chest up and back. Keep your elbows bent and close to your sides.

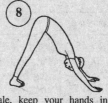

8

Exhale, keep your hands in the same place, straighten your arms, and lift your hips as high as possible while placing your feet flat on the floor.

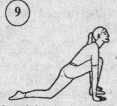

9

Inhale and, keeping your hands in the same place, drop your hips and stretch your left leg back. Drop your left knee to the ground, keeping your arms straight.

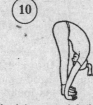

10

Exhale, bring your left foot forward, and lift your hips up. Keep your hands on the ground and slide them toward you so that they are flat on the ground on either side of your feet, with your toes and fingers aligned.

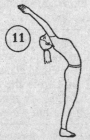

11

Inhale and stretch your arms out over your head. Roll your hips forward and arch back from the waist, pushing your head back.

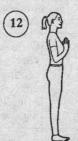

12

Stand up straight, shoulders back, feet together, arms hanging loosely at your sides. Exhale as you bring your hands together in front of you.

Exercise	How it helps
Brisk walking	Good weight-bearing exercise for the bones. Can be fitted in easily with your lifestyle. Healthy exercise for the heart, muscles, and lungs.
Jogging/ running	Good weight-bearing exercise for the bones. Can be fitted in at any time. Helps to release euphoria-linked endorphins and helps to lower cholesterol and prevent heart disease. Be careful of your joints if you are running on concrete: buy well-cushioned running shoes. And try not to run in a traffic-polluted area.
Re- bounding	Uses a small "trampoline" at home, so you can do this exercise at any time. Gentle on the joints and a good weight-bearing exercise. Also good for the heart, lungs and circulation. There are books and videos available on this.
Racket sports	Good weight-bearing activity. Sociable exercise, so can be more motivating than exercising on your own. Be careful not to put your racket arm under too much strain, producing a negative effect.
Swimming	Good aerobic activity for the heart and lungs. Easy on the joints but not weight-bearing. Osteopaths are concerned about the effect on the neck and back from the head being kept out of the water, so try to swim with your whole body in one line.
Dancing	A sociable, fun activity. Good for weight-bearing and also excellent for coordination which can prevent accidents at the menopause.

Exercise	How it helps
Yoga	A good all-around activity. Improves flexibility, suppleness, and breathing. Excellent for the mind and body, as it can help to reduce stress and give you tools to keep you calm.
Cycling	A good exercise that can be done on an exercise bike or as a social activity. Excellent for muscle tone and strengthening. Good exercise for pumping blood into the vaginal area.
Aerobic exercises	These are energetic movements performed to music. Good for the bones, heart, and circulation. You can join a class which makes it more social, especially if you go with a friend. You can also use a video at home. Take things gradually at first, and find the right level for yourself.
T'ai chi/ Qi gong	These are Eastern forms of exercise which have mental as well as physical benefits. They are like a moving meditation. They need to taught by an experienced practitioner and then can be practiced on your own. In China, the workforce of a company will perform these *en masse* before the start of a working day.
Alexander Technique	This is not an exercise but a way of helping you to keep your posture as nature intended. Only the minimum of effort is needed to produce a movement. As the menopause takes place, there is the possibility of kyphosis (dowager's hump), so any help with our posture will be an advantage.

support their weight better and maintain their shape. Here are two exercises to try:

1. Stand 2ft. (60cm.) away from a wall and place your hands flat against it, 1ft. (30cm.) wider than your shoulders. Breathe in, bend your elbows, and lean toward the wall. Try to touch the wall with your nose, keeping your back flat and your legs straight, as if you were doing a vertical push-up. Hold for a few seconds, then push away. Repeat five times.
2. Bend your elbows and press your palms together as if in a prayer position but with your elbows sticking out. Press your palms together as firmly as possible. Hold for a few seconds and then relax. Repeat five times.

How old would you be if you didn't know how old you were?

Our biological age can differ from our chronological age. The difference, scientists believe, is due to a number of things including our genetic inheritance as well as lifestyle factors such as diet, smoking, drinking, and exercise.

This test, reproduced by kind permission of the British newspaper the *Daily Mail* from an article by Andrew Willson, April 1995, can give an approximate indication of your biological age.

Circle the number after each of your answers, and add them up to give a total score:

1. *Do you or have you ever smoked?*
   No, never   1
   Once or twice   3
   A few a day   4
   A pack a day   5

2. *Do you drink? (1 unit is about 4fl.oz. (125ml.) of wine or 10fl.oz. (285ml.) of beer or about 1fl.oz. (25ml.) of spirits)*
   No, never   3

1–2 units a day	1
3–4 units a day	4
More than this	5

3. *How many servings of high-fat foods (fried food, dairy products, etc.) do you have a day?*

None	1
Two or three	3
Three to six	4
More than this	5

4. *How often do you eat red meat?*

Never	1
Three to five times a week	4
More than this	5

5. *How often do you eat fish?*

Never	5
Once a week	3
Twice a week	2
Three or more	1

6. *How many servings or pieces of fruit and vegetables do you eat each day?*

None	5
One or two	3
Three or four	2
Five or more	1

7. *Do you sunbathe or work outdoors without adequate protection from the sun's rays?*

Yes, all the time	5
Once or twice a year	4
Never	1

8. *With your thumb and forefinger, pinch a piece of skin on the back of your hand and hold in this position for five seconds. Release and then count how many seconds it takes for the skin to resume its original position.*

Age 40s–50s		*Over 60s*	
One second	1	Five or less seconds	1
Two seconds	2	Six to ten seconds	2

Three or four seconds	3	Eleven to fifteen seconds	3
Five to ten seconds	4	Sixteen to twenty seconds	4
More than ten seconds	5	More than twenty-one seconds	5

9. *Examine one of your fingernails under a bright light. Turn it slowly so you can see the texture of the nail.*

	Age 40+	Age 50+	Age 60+
No ridging or discoloration	1	1	1
Slight ridging	1	1	1
Noticeable ridging	5	3	3
Very noticeable ridging	5	3	3
Severe and extreme ridging	5	5	5

10. *How many hours of exercise do you do a week?*

	Age 40–50	Age 60+
None	4	3
One	2	2
More than one	1	1

11. *Sit on the floor, extend your right leg straight in front of you, and place the heel of your left foot against your right thigh. Then stretch your right arm as far as it will go towards your toes. How far can you stretch?*

	Age 40–50	Age 60+
Your wrist on your toes	1	1
Your fingertips on your toes	2	1
Your fingers on your ankle	3	2
Your fingers on your sock line	4	3

12. *Sit on a bottom step with your legs stretched straight out in front of you, with your heels on the ground, and your toes pointing upward. Move your body so that your hands rest on the top of the stair and gently ease yourself down, bending your elbows until they are at*

90 degrees. Now try to push yourself back up. How many of these can you do easily?

Age 40s		Age 50s		Over 60s	
Seven+ lifts	1	Six+ lifts	1	Five+ lifts	1
Six	3	Five	3	Four	3
Five or fewer	5	Four or fewer	5	Three or fewer	5

13. *For this test you will need an 8-in.- (20cm.) -high step or box and a wristwatch with a second hand. Step up with your left foot, then your right, then step back down with your left and back down with your right. Do twenty complete steps per minute and continue for three minutes. After the three minutes are up, wait fifteen seconds and then take your pulse, count for fifteen seconds, multiply this by four to get the total number of beats per minute, and write this down. Then check your figure against your age group.*

40s		Over 50s	
100 beats per minute	1	100 beats per minute	1
145 beats per minute	3	150 beats per minute	3
175 beats per minute	5	175 beats per minute	5

14. *How would you rate your general outlook on life?*

You can't bear to get out of bed in the morning	5
Generally pessimistic	4
Content	3
You try to look on the bright side	2
You see each day as a fresh challenge	1

15. *How do you react in stressful situations?*

Panic and fall to pieces	5
Get angry and lose your temper	4
Take a couple of deep breaths but still don't know how to deal with the problems	3
Calmly assess the situation and try to solve it	2
Thrive on stress and use it positively	1

How did you score?

Up to 15

You could be between five and ten years younger than your chronological age. Carry on with your healthy diet and life-style, and continue exercising.

Between 16 and 31

You could be between two and five years younger than your actual age, depending on whether you are closer to the higher or lower score. If you want to improve your score, look at those areas where you scored 2 or above and see what changes you can make.

Between 32 and 47

If you scored at the lower end of this category, the test indicates that you are biologically a couple of years younger than your chronological age. If you are near the score of 47, your chronological and biological age are almost the same. Look at the questions where you circled 3 or above and see what changes you can make.

Between 48 and 63

Scoring near the 48 mark means that your body is likely to be a few years older than average for your age. If your score is nearer 63, then you could be up to five years older than your chronological age. Follow the recommendations in this book and make some definite changes.

Between 64 and 79

You are getting old before your time. A score near 64 suggests you may be at least five years older than your chronological age, whereas a score nearer 79 means you could be up to ten years older. Look at your lifestyle; it is never too late to change, and our bodies are very resilient.

Staying active, mobile, and fit is extremely important at the menopause. The benefits are numerous, but it does require some effort and organization. Combined with sensible diet and nutrition, exercise is one of the most important things a woman can do to help herself through the menopause. Quite how important, we may never know. The vast majority of medical research is devoted to finding "cures" for "symptoms." The pharmaceutical industry wants products to sell. It is not terribly interested in discovering the fact that exercise may prevent or relieve menopausal symptoms, which is why the benefits of exercise are not examined more closely or promoted more aggressively.

Sex is good for you, too

As we have seen, exercise can help your sex life. But sex itself is good for you and stimulates the hormones. Sex releases tension and calms you down. It helps to boost the immune system and to relieve headaches and arthritis. A massive research project involving 55,000 people conducted by the Institute for Advanced Study of Human Sexuality in San Francisco found that those who had a satisfying sex life were physically healthier and more relaxed than those who reported an unfulfilling sex life. Ted McIlvenna, President of the Institute, was even quoted as saying, "Sex is perhaps the best preventive and healing medicine there is." That may be a bit of an exaggeration, but it makes the point that sex is important for a balanced healthy life. The fact is that sex releases the brain chemicals known as endorphins that make us feel content and happy with the world. Perking up the libido is one of the supposed benefits of taking Hormone Replacement Therapy. But there is no real evidence that changing hormone levels have any effect on a woman's sexuality at all. What may undermine it, however, is the notion that the menopause is some kind of crisis, that when the biological clock starts to chime, a woman inevitably becomes less attractive. This is rubbish.

But it can adversely affect women's sexual confidence and attitudes, particularly when every single problem you have is put down to "your hormones."

In fact the menopause and beyond should be seen as a time for greater sexual enjoyment. Children are no longer a tie, and you don't have to worry about contraception. Some women have an increased sexual drive at this time. That's because the level of testosterone, the male hormone we all have in our bodies, becomes proportionately higher. The famous anthropologist Margaret Mead called this "post menopausal zest." Postmenopausal women can have up to twenty times the amount of testosterone as pre-menopausal women. How's that for the "hormonal deficit" we are all supposed to be suffering from?

Testosterone is the hormone linked to drive, motivation, and assertiveness. Perhaps this explains why, in traditional cultures, older women are regarded as counselors, leaders, and lawmakers.

Contraception

As a rule of thumb, you should wait for two clear period-free years before abandoning contraception if your menopause starts before the age of fifty. If you were over fifty when it started, a year free of periods is considered safe.

Vaginal dryness

Besides the Kegel exercises (see page 197) and the vitamin E supplementation I have already recommended, there are some lubricants available. One good one is called Astroglide. It's a gel that closely resembles our own body's lubricant and is mildly acidic like our own secretions. Many vaginal lubricants sold over the counter alter the balance of the bacteria in the vagina designed to protect us from infection. But Astroglide is water-soluble, non-hormonal, and safe to use with condoms if you are still having periods and need a contraceptive.

Sexual satisfaction

There is no reason why sex should not be as satisfying now as at any other time of your life. And several good reasons why it should actually be better. Women have always taken longer to become aroused than men, and when we are young the difference can be quite striking. A man in his twenties can achieve orgasm within two to five minutes, whereas his partner may take twenty minutes. As a man gets older he needs longer to reach an orgasm, so the timing, in theory, becomes more compatible. Sex can take longer, and intercourse may not necessarily be the main focus. You may have sex less often than in your twenties, but it can be a deeper, more satisfying experience. The truth is that the aging process has an effect on both men and women—and the so-called "male menopause" may pose much more of a real problem in sexual terms for your partner. Women may worry about their attractiveness but many middle-aged men become very concerned about their sexual performance. Both partners may need to make adjustments at the menopause. Communication and honesty are the key and can prevent misunderstandings and resentment from building up between you and your partner. By communicating honestly about what we like and don't like, changing positions if one we have always used makes us uncomfortable, and taking the steps recommended to counteract any physical changes, there is no reason why sex should not continue to be thoroughly enjoyable.

The biggest sexual problem for many women has nothing to do with hormones, vaginal dryness, or anything else that can be explained medically. It is boredom. Many women have stayed in a relationship for the sake of their children. Other couples are happy enough but find that passion and excitement have just fizzled out. A patient once said to me that HRT was wonderful. Not Hormone Replacement Therapy, she said, but Husband Replacement Therapy. Once the children have grown up and left home, a couple may find they just don't have very much in common anymore. This can expose weaknesses in a relationship. This is one reason why women feel they have reached an important turning point in their lives. Even if they are happy in a relationship, they are conscious of the fact that they have put their children and husbands first for as far back as they can remember.

CHAPTER 12

Tests at the menopause

There are a number of tests available that are worth having at the menopause. These tests can let you know what condition your body is in now. They can tell you what vitamin and mineral deficiencies and heavy toxic metal excesses you may have and let you know the condition of your bones and how well your digestive system is functioning. They can also help you assess what you might need in the form of food supplements in order to bring your body back into balance and optimum health, helping to prevent future problems from arising.

Hormone tests (blood and saliva)

A simple blood test can measure your hormone levels and determine whether you are in the menopause. Your FSH (follicle stimulating hormone) tends to rise dramatically during the menopause, and if it appears high this would indicate that you are menopausal.

Another simple and very effective non-invasive test can be carried out on the saliva to measure the levels of the two major classes of ovarian hormones, estrogen and progesterone, at the menopause. Using a specially designed kit, you collect a sample of your own saliva, seal it in the container supplied, and send it off directly to the laboratory for analysis. The results include measurements of your current levels of estriol, estradiol, progestrone, DHEA, and testosterone.

I feel that a hormone test is important if you are considering HRT, as one woman I saw who had been put on hormones now has a level of estrogen that her hospital considers too high. She has been told to come off the drug and wait for the level to drop. It is possible and very likely that her estrogen level was adequate before she was given the hormones, and the additional hormones may well have caused an imbalance.

Personalized supplement and nutritional program (questionnaire)

Your health depends on a whole range of factors such as diet, lifestyle, stress, age, etc. With modern life being so busy and stressful, it may not be possible for you to eat as well as you would like, and much of the food you do eat is likely to be deficient in the vitamins and minerals needed to keep your body healthy and well balanced.

Your health also depends on how well you absorb and digest the nutrients you do eat. Problems such as lack of energy, insomnia, headaches, depression, mood swings, anxiety, etc., can be traced directly to deficiencies of specific vitamins and minerals.

Vitamins and minerals work in balance with one another. It is because of this that it is vital you take the right ones in the right amounts, in the right combination, and at the right times.

It is possible to have a personalized supplement and nutritional program designed specifically according to your symptoms and lifestyle factors. If you complete a comprehensive questionnaire that explores your lifestyle, symptoms, and dietary profile, the vitamin and mineral levels present in your body can be checked and assessed for deficiencies. When analyzed, the results are sent to you in a detailed report showing the 12 vitamins (A, D, E, C, B1, B2, B3, B5, B6, B12, folic acid, and biotin) and 7 minerals (calcium, magnesium, zinc, manganese, chromium, selenium, and iron) and the essential fatty acids you need to take, and in what quantities you need these in order to bring your body back into balance and optimum health. The report also includes dietary targets to help you function at your peak levels of energy and health.

At the end of three months, you are reassessed after filling in the questionnaire again. The results are compared with your original ones to see how your levels have changed, and your supplement program is then adjusted according to any changes found.

This is an excellent test to determine what supplements would be of most benefit for you now according to your symptoms, diet, and lifestyle and to monitor your progress over time.

Osteoporosis risk evaluation test (urine)

Many women at the menopause are rightly concerned about osteoporosis. It is one of the main reasons why they choose HRT. But you should not feel pressured into taking HRT just because of the fear of osteoporosis. There is now a safe way to find out what your bone health is like.

A special non-invasive osteoporosis risk evaluation urine test has recently been developed in the United States (it is also available in Britain). By taking this test you can discover the condition your bones are in now and assess any potential risk of osteoporosis. It shows you what is happening biochemically in your bones and gives you a dynamic picture of bone turnover (this is when bone formation does not keep up with bone loss) and a prediction of the risk of future loss rather than just a one-off snapshot measure in a bone density scan. This test is reported to be just as accurate as bone scanning in identifying those at risk. It measures pyridinium and deoxypyridinium, two collagen cross links, which change and are excreted in the urine as the bone breaks down. With this test you are in control, you take the urine sample yourself, and there is no exposure to potentially harmful X-rays.

If your bone health is good, you are in the wonderful position of being able to work on prevention naturally with good diet, supplements, and exercise and to monitor your bones to make sure they are staying healthy. If you are losing bone, at least you know what is happening and can get the most appropriate treatment.

Mineral analysis (hair)

With this test you can find out what deficiencies of minerals and excesses of heavy toxic metals are present in your body and have a personalized supplement program designed specifically according to your own biochemical profile. Your hair sample is tested and analyzed in a laboratory, and from the results it is possible to assess your levels of calcium, magnesium, zinc, selenium, manganese, chromium, and nickel and identify any deficiencies present. It also provides valuable information on your levels of heavy toxic metals such as mercury, aluminum, lead, cadmium, and arsenic. These are all shown in the form of a graph (see next page) so you can see how far your levels differ from the norm.

This test can tell you a lot about what may be going on in your body. I have seen a number of women with a high calcium level in their hair, for instance, which indicates there may be a high calcium turnover in the bone, suggesting they might have problems keeping their calcium levels stable. After the results of the test, any deficiencies can be supplemented and action can be taken to reduce the levels of any heavy toxic metals. An osteoporosis risk evaluation urine test can also be used in combination with the hair results to identify cases of high bone turnover. The hair can be then be re-tested in three months' time to confirm that the levels are back to normal or whether the supplements need adjusting according to your new condition.

It is also wise to have the hair test done in conjunction with the personal supplement and nutritional program. By comparing your biochemical and lifestyle results, a more comprehensive profile of your overall condition is achieved. Compare the charts opposite.

Results of hair mineral analysis test before treatment

(ALL RESULTS IN PARTS PER MILLION)

	REFERENCE RANGE	RESULTS	|	LOW	|	REFERENCE RANGE	|	HIGH	|	
CALCIUM	200 - 600	538								Ca
MAGNESIUM	30 - 95	27								Mg
PHOSPHORUS*	100 - 210	117								P
SODIUM*	90 - 340	514								Na
POTASSIUM*	50 - 120	67								K
IRON*	20 - 60	30								Fe
COPPER	10 - 40	27								Cu
ZINC	150 - 240	137								Zn
CHROMIUM	0.60 - 1.50	0.76								Cr
MANGANESE	1.0 - 2.6	1.1								Mn
SELENIUM	1.5 - 4.0	1.5								Se
NICKEL	0.40 - 1.40	0.67								Ni
COBALT*	0.10 - 0.70	0.24								Co

* Clinical significance of hair concentration of asterisked elements has not been established.

	ACCEPT	RAISED	TOXIC	RESULT	|	ACCEPTABLE	|	RAISED	|	TOXIC	|	
LEAD	<15.0	15.0 - 40.0	>40.0	4.1								Pb
MERCURY	<2.0	2.0 - 5.0	>5.0	0.37								Hg
CADMIUM	<0.5	0.5 - 2.0	>2.0	0.53								Cd
ARSENIC	<2.0	2.0 - 5.0	>5.0	0.24								As
ALUMINIUM	<10.0	10.0 - 25.0	>25.0	2.1								Al

Results of hair mineral analysis test after treatment

(ALL RESULTS IN PARTS PER MILLION)

	REFERENCE RANGE	RESULTS	:	LOW	:	REFERENCE RANGE	:	HIGH	:	
CALCIUM	200 - 600	516								Ca
MAGNESIUM	30 - 95	46								Mg
PHOSPHORUS*	100 - 210	170								P
SODIUM*	90 - 340	220								Na
POTASSIUM*	50 - 120	78								K
IRON*	20 - 60	21								Fe
COPPER	10 - 40	27								Cu
ZINC	150 - 240	193								Zn
CHROMIUM	0.60 - 1.50	0.71								Cr
MANGANESE	1.0 - 2.6	1.4								Mn
SELENIUM	1.5 - 4.0	2.2								Se
NICKEL	0.40 - 1.40	0.71								Ni
COBALT*	0.10 - 0.70	0.19								Co

* Clinical significance of hair concentration of asterisked elements has not been established.

	ACCEPT	RAISED	TOXIC	RESULT	:	ACCEPTABLE	:	RAISED	:	TOXIC	:	
LEAD	<15.0	15.0 - 40.0	>40.0	3.9								Pb
MERCURY	<2.0	2.0 - 5.0	>5.0	0.40								Hg
CADMIUM	<0.5	0.5 - 2.0	>2.0	0.17								Cd
ARSENIC	<2.0	2.0 - 5.0	>5.0	0.16								As
ALUMINIUM	<10.0	10.0 - 25.0	>25.0	1.6								Al

The two hair mineral analysis charts above show the difference before and after taking food supplements. In the first chart the patient has lower levels of magnesium, zinc, and selenium, and her cadmium level is too high as a result of smoking. In the second chart, after following an appropriate supplement program, her mineral levels are back to normal and the cadmium is reduced (she gave up smoking, too).

Food allergy tests (blood)

There are now available a number of blood tests that can reveal the foods that you are allergic to that are believed to trigger symptoms such as weight gain, bloating, aching joints, fatigue, stuffy nose, skin problems, migraine headaches, asthma, and digestive disorders. Allergies to some foods in certain people appear to make the body retain water—and gain weight. Some people are aware that they are allergic to certain foods—the reaction is immediate and usually dramatic, like getting a rash after eating strawberries. But many of us suffer more subtle reactions. People who become overweight, for instance, may have an allergic reaction to certain foods that compels them to eat beyond their energy requirements. Ironically, it is the foods to which we are allergic that we often crave, as if we had a mild addiction.

If your body's immune system is "fighting" some of the foods you are eating, it is likely that it will be operating less effectively and will be less able to get rid of any toxins and excess weight. These kinds of allergies can now be identified.

There are two main blood tests for food allergies, the cytotoxic test and the IgG antibody test.

Cytotoxic test

This test measures the reaction of your white blood cells when brought into contact with foods and chemicals. The white cells may react by becoming smaller or larger or by disintegrating. The test shows if your body is "seeing" certain foods as toxins and then producing an immune system reaction to them, causing you to experience certain allergic symptoms.

ELISA IgG Test

The ELISA test (enzyme linked immuno-sorbent assay) is a very sensitive way of testing for food allergies.

This test measures the IgG antibody reaction to certain foods. When your food is not being digested properly (see "Leaky gut" below), food particles can leak out into the bloodstream. Instead of your body seeing these particles as food, it views them as toxins and sends out IgG antibodies to cope with them. When there are too many, they clump together and get deposited in the soft tissues around the body in the joints, muscles, skin, brain, etc. This can cause symptoms such as weight gain, fatigue, water retention, pain, and inflammation, to name but a few. By measuring the IgG antibody reaction to certain foods it is possible to find out which foods you should avoid in order to prevent any "allergic" reactions you may be experiencing.

By using either of the above two blood allergy tests first to identify and then to eliminate the foods your body is reacting to, you will start to remove the cause of the inflammatory conditions and are likely to notice an improvement that may be dramatic.

With these tests you are sent a special kit that enables your doctor or a nurse to take a small quantity of blood. This is sent to the laboratory, and after it has been analyzed you are sent an extensive personalized report showing

- a list of foods that are highly reactive for you and those that are borderline and also those that are non-reactive for you,
- recommendations of how to implement food changes and how to reintroduce the reactive/borderline foods safely at a later date.

I have had excellent results with these tests. I am told that one woman lost 13 pounds (6kg.) in four weeks after taking a test and following the recommendations. Others have reported significant reductions in their symptoms.

Both types of test have been used to identify clinical problems, and both of them have had scientific research published on them which supports these findings.[1]

Leaky gut (urine)

Tracking down the foods to which you are sensitive is solving only half the problem. Why have you developed this sensitivity in the first place? What happens when you reintroduce the offending foods to your diet? The answer lies in the state of your intestines, your gut, and its capacity to process food properly. Food allergies are often the symptom that all is not well. This is very important at the menopause, because if you are not absorbing nutrients efficiently, you can become deficient in vital vitamins and minerals. All food you eat must be broken down by the digestive system, passed into the bloodstream and dealt with successfully by your body's lymph system. If the food is not broken down properly, your body "sees" this normal food as an antigen, a toxin, and sets up an immune system reaction to deal with it. At the same time, this undigested food is sitting around fermenting and putrefying. This unhealthy environment in the gut allows yeasts like candida to overrun. We all have candida in our gut, but it is controlled by other "good" bacteria. In an unhealthy gut environment, however, it proliferates out of control. Large spaces can develop between the cells in the gut wall, and food molecules can then pass into the bloodstream. This is leaky gut or intestinal permeability. So initially it is important to stop eating the offending foods, which will help to alleviate the symptoms and make you feel better. Then the whole environment of the gut needs to be healed as well, in order to get the intestinal bacteria back in balance again so that you can stay healthy and prevent the symptoms from recurring.

This condition has only recently become widely recognized, and there is now a very effective non-invasive urine test available to assess intestinal permeability. Two urine samples are required for this test. The first one is a pre-test sample and the second one is taken six hours after you drink a special liquid which contains two marker molecules. When the samples are analyzed, the amount of the marker molecules detected by the laboratory will give a strong indication as to how permeable (i.e. how leaky) your gut is. Once you have this information, you can then decide the best course of action to take to heal.

There are, of course, other tests that can help at the menopause, but lack of space prevents explanation of all of them. The ones mentioned above are the ones I use the most and from which I have always obtained the best results.

If you are concerned about your health and the symptoms you may be experiencing, these tests are important for you to help find out what condition your body is in now. Only after undergoing them can you make an informed decision as to the best program of treatment you should undertake to bring yourself back to optimum health. You can then monitor your progress over time by being retested every three to six months and adjusting your treatment according to your current state of health.

CHAPTER 13

Menopause meal plans

I have covered all the good foods to include in your diet at the menopause in the chapter on nutrition, but how do you put this into practice when you have not only yourself to feed but also the family? I have given a choice of meals for breakfast, lunch, and dinner with recipes assuming that you will probably be cooking for the family (either partner and/or children) only once a day and able to choose your own food for breakfast and lunch. If you are at home during the week, this makes the choice of food much easier, but many of us are away from the house and are restricted by the choices we have, and I have tried to take this into account.

Most of us do not have a lot of time for preparing meals except when we are expecting guests, so meals on a day-to-day basis need to be quick and easy to prepare and yet healthy and nutritious. I have included simple recipes and also more complicated and time-consuming ones. Those with a variety of different ingredients can be adapted to suit your time and what you already have available.

Aim to keep the foundation of your food healthful, so that when you are eating out it will be no big deal if you include other less healthful foods. In a couple of the recipes you will see ingredients like cream and coconut cream (both saturated fats) which are added in small quantities whereas the majority of the rest of the ingredients are healthful.

I do not eat red meat or chicken, so I have excluded these from the menus. You are welcome to substitute these for fish in the appropriate recipes.

In your own favorite dishes you can substitute whole-wheat flour for white flour, free-range eggs for ordinary eggs, soy milk for animal milk, and clear honey or maple syrup for sugar (using the same quantity). Remember: if a food is described as sugar-free, this does not mean that it is not sweet, and there are a number of cookbooks with recipes for desserts made from naturally sweet ingredients instead of sugar. If you suspect you may be allergic to wheat, you can substitute spelt for wheat in any of the recipes. Spelt is related to wheat, but people who are normally allergic to gluten seem to tolerate it better.

With the scientific knowledge we have of the effects of different foods on our health and hormones, it is wise to emphasize foods such as soy, vegetable oils, oily fish, nuts, seeds, fruits (especially the strong-colored ones), and vegetables. Sesame seeds are valuable for their calcium content and can be used just as the seeds or as tahini (sesame butter). I have also included the mixture of cider vinegar and honey in a number of recipes, as this helps to increase calcium absorption (see Chapter 7, page 135).

Soy, with its weak estrogenic action, is a valuable food to add at the menopause, and this may well be the first time you have used it. It comes in many forms, as soybeans, tofu (beancurd), soy milk, soy sauce (the best one being wheat-free tamari), miso, and tempeh. It is easier to get used to soy by adding it to your diet gradually. Soy sauce is the first form to try; it gives a delicious flavor to stir-fries, etc. Next try substituting soy milk for animal milk in a sauce, then in a hot drink, and then on cereals. Tempeh is definitely an acquired taste and not always easy to find, so it would be best to concentrate on the other soy products.

Breakfasts

Granola   Choose a good sugar-free granola or muesli.
Oatmeal   Buy organic, if possible, and cook it with water. Top with linseeds or sunflower or sesame seeds, or mix in a teaspoon of sugar-free jam or a dash of pure maple syrup. When using small seeds such as linseeds or sesame seeds, it is best to crack the seed

in a grinder or pestle and mortar before you eat it, otherwise it can pass through you undigested.

Cornflakes Buy sugar-free cornflakes, which are usually sweetened with apple juice, and have them with organic soy milk or organic cows' or goats' milk.

Whole-wheat toast with sugar-free jam Avoid diabetic preserves which contain sorbitol; choose only those made with pure fruit such as Polaner All Fruit or St. Dalfour.

Natural live yogurt with your choice of fruit Try bananas, peaches, or strawberries.

Dried fruit soaked overnight When you buy dried fruit, choose brands that do not have sulfur dioxide added. It is used to preserve the color of apricots, for example, but they taste just as delicious without it.

Other cereals Shredded Wheat, Puffed Rice, or Puffed Wheat, with organic soy milk or organic cows' or goats' milk. Or you can make your own cereal:

CRUNCHY OAT CEREAL

Serves 4

4 tablespoons clear honey or maple syrup
8 tablespoons corn oil
4½ cups (450g.) rolled oats
1⅓ cups (100g.) shredded coconut
⅔ cup (100g.) raisins
1 cup (100g.) roasted nuts (almonds, cashews, peanuts, etc.)

Combine the honey or maple syrup and oil and pour into a large bowl.

Add the oats and coconut, and combine well so that they are completely covered with the honey and oil mixture.

Bake in a low oven for approximately an hour until the oats are golden and crisp.

Mix in the raisins and nuts and leave to cool, then store in an airtight jar.

Lunches

If you are working and have a limited choice of food for lunch, you could have sandwiches a couple of days a week and take something slightly more substantial on the others.

Sandwiches Choose whole-wheat bread. Whole-wheat pitas can also make a change from sliced bread. Suggestions for fillings:

- tahini and freshly sliced apple
- mashed avocado with a sprinkling of sunflower seeds
- tuna and lettuce
- egg and watercress
- avocado and lettuce

- hummus and lettuce
- bean sprouts and tahini
- tofu mashed with a little miso and lettuce
- miso, tahini, lettuce, and a squeeze of lemon

Baked potato with corn/tuna/mixed salad/hummus

Homemade soups Try Carrot and Cashew (see page 232) or lentil (this could be taken to work in a thermos), or buy a canned soup with good ingredients, such as Health Valley.

Smoked mackerel and mixed salad

Leftovers Some lunches, such as soups, can be made from leftovers from your meal of the night before. This will cut down on preparation. Leftover vegetables and rice can also be quickly stir-fried for an appetizing lunch.

Or try the following recipes:

TUNA FISH AND BROWN RICE SALAD

Serves 4

This is a quick and easy lunchtime recipe because you can use leftover rice. It can be prepared the night before and kept in the fridge to take to work.

1 tablespoon cider vinegar
3 tablespoons olive oil
1 teaspoon mustard (optional)
Juice of ½ lemon
1½ cups (230g.) cooked long or short-grain brown rice,
organic if possible
7-oz. (200g.) can tuna fish, drained (you can now buy tuna
in spring water)
A few drops of soy sauce
2in. (5cm.) cucumber, finely chopped
1 tablespoon fresh parsley, chopped

In a screw-top jar, combine the vinegar, oil, mustard (if using), and lemon juice, and then shake until mixed thoroughly.

Place the cooked rice in a fairly large bowl and pour over the oil and vinegar mixture.

Flake the tuna and add to the rice.

Add the soy sauce, cucumber, and parsley and mix thoroughly.

Avocado Dip

Makes enough for 4

This is delicious as a filling for pita or as a dip with raw carrots, celery and cucumber, or tortilla chips. If I am short of time or I have not thought far enough ahead (as is often the case), I skip the eggs, which are supposed to be hard-boiled. I like it equally well with or without the eggs. This recipe uses both cider vinegar and honey, which enable calcium to be better utilized. Choose either a good soy mayonnaise (these are often egg-free) or a good "ordinary" mayonnaise made entirely with natural ingredients.

1 tablespoon cider vinegar
Juice of 1 lemon
6 tablespoons mayonnaise
1 tablespoon fresh parsley, finely chopped
3 hard-boiled eggs
1 ripe avocado

1 teaspoon clear honey or maple syrup
Sea salt and freshly ground black pepper (optional)

This is easy: just put all the ingredients in the blender and turn it on.

STIR-FRY VEGETABLE NOODLES

Serves 4

This recipe is very quick and easy to prepare. It can be served by itself for a light meal or as an accompaniment to broiled fish or chicken. Other vegetables may be used, so long as they can be shredded so that the cooking is quick, e.g. celeriac, cabbage, or even bean sprouts and thinly sliced water chestnuts.

1 tablespoon extra-virgin olive oil
1 tablespoon fresh root ginger, finely chopped
2 garlic cloves, finely chopped
Cooked Chinese fresh egg noodles
Grated zucchini
Grated carrots

Heat the oil in a wok or heavy frying pan, until slightly smoking. Add the ginger and garlic, and cook until lightly browned, stirring constantly. Then add the noodles and vegetables, in quantity to suit your taste, and continue stirring until cooked, about 5 minutes.

Soups

MISO SOUP

Serves 1

Miso soup is a traditional Japanese dish which is served every day. Miso is fermented soybean paste; because of the fermentation process it contains enzymes beneficial for digestion in the same way that yogurt does. It also contains compounds that are important at the menopause.

I have found miso soup to be an acquired taste. Miso can be used as a seasoning for casseroles and other thicker soups such as lentil or vegetable, and this is an easier way to introduce it into your meals.

33cm. (13in.) strip dry wakame seaweed
1 onion, thinly sliced
300ml. (1¼ cup) of water
1 tablespoon miso (or to taste)
Grated fresh root ginger, or chopped green onions or parsley to garnish

Rinse the wakame under cold water to remove excess sea salt and to clean it. Then cut into ½-in. (1cm.) pieces.

Place the wakame and onion in a saucepan and add the water. Bring to the boil, place the lid on the pan and simmer for about 20 minutes. Reduce the heat of the soup so that it is very low and not bubbling.

In a small bowl combine the miso and a small quantity of the broth from the soup. Stir until the miso is a smooth paste.

Add the miso paste to the soup. Once the miso is added to the soup, the heat should be kept very low; otherwise the beneficial enzymes in the miso could be destroyed. Simmer for 3–5 minutes and serve, garnished with grated ginger, or chopped green onions or parsley.

This soup can be varied by adding in sliced carrots and/or celery while it is cooking and watercress at the very end of cooking.

CARROT AND CASHEW SOUP

Serves 6

3 pints (1.4 liter) leftover vegetable stock or water
3lb. (1.5kg.) carrots, chopped
1 teaspoon sea salt
1¼ cup (150g.) chopped onions
¾ cups (100g.) unsalted, unroasted cashews
3 garlic cloves, crushed
2 tablespoons olive oil

1¼ pint (600ml.) soy milk
1 tablespoon fresh root ginger, grated
Black pepper (optional)
Parsley, yogurt, or toasted cashews to garnish

Add the stock or water to the carrots and salt in a saucepan, and bring to the boil. Cover and simmer for 15 minutes. Meanwhile, in another pan, sauté the onions, cashews, and garlic in the olive oil until the onions are translucent and soft.

Put the contents of the two saucepans into a blender, and purée until very smooth. Return the purée to a saucepan and add the soy milk, ginger, and black pepper (if using). Garnish with parsley, yogurt, or toasted cashews.

SOYBEAN AND VEGETABLE SOUP

Serves 6

1 cup (200g.) uncooked soybean or canned soybeans
1 large onion, chopped
1 garlic clove, chopped
1 carrot, chopped
1 stick celery, chopped
1 tablespoon olive oil
2 pints (950ml.) water or vegetable stock
1 teaspoon dried sage
½ teaspoon each dried tarragon, dried marjoram, and
caraway seeds
Pinch of sea salt or miso

If using uncooked beans, cover with unsalted water and soak overnight.

Sauté the onion, garlic, carrot, and celery in the heated oil. Discard the soaking water from the beans and add them to the vegetables with the water or stock. Add the herbs. Cook for 1½ hours, or 30 minutes in a pressure cooker. (Or about 10–15 minutes if using canned beans.) Season with salt or miso.

Main meals

EASY WAYS TO COOK BROWN RICE

Brown rice provides more nutrients than white rice because it is a whole food. Use it in recipes where you would previously have used white rice. Because rice grains are small, they can absorb more pesticides than, say, a carrot, so it is advisable to buy organic brown rice. The usual rule of thumb is to have long-grain brown rice in summer and the heartier short-grain in winter, but this choice can also depend on the dish you are making. For lighter dishes use long-grain, for heavier dishes short-grain. For Indian dishes, I recommend brown basmati rice, or white basmati for a change.

I always cook more brown rice than I need for a meal, because leftover rice, once cool, will keep for several days in the refrigerator and can be used for quick lunches or dinners. To heat up leftover rice, either sauté in a little oil or add tamari (wheat-free soya sauce) to taste, or steam the rice in a small-holed vegetable steamer over boiling water.

BOILED BROWN RICE

1 cup (200g.) brown rice
2 cups (470 ml.) water
Pinch sea salt

Wash the rice and place in a heavy saucepan. Add the water and salt, cover with a lid, and bring to the boil. Once it is boiling, lower the heat and simmer for about 40 minutes or until the water has been absorbed.

BAKED BROWN RICE

If I know that I am going to be short of time in the evening, I set the time on the oven and bake the rice.

The proportions are the same as for boiled rice (above), and I set it to cook for 1 hour at 400°F (200°C). At the same time I may also bake some parsnips or onions. Another useful and delicious vegetable to cook at the same time as the rice is squash. Put the whole squash (butternut or acorn) on a baking sheet and brush with a light covering of olive oil to prevent it from cracking. This takes the same length of time to cook as the rice.

PRESSURE-COOKED BROWN RICE

I find this way of cooking really easy. Once the cooker is sealed and I have set the timer, I can do other things, because I don't feel I have to keep checking it.

2 cups (400g.) brown rice
3 cups (700 ml.) water
Pinch of sea salt

Put the rice and water in the pressure cooker with the salt, and slowly bring up to pressure. Once the pressure is up, lower the heat and place a steel mesh heat deflector under the pan (this stops the rice from sticking). Cook for approximately 30–35 minutes with the pressure still gently up.

When the rice is cooked, turn the heat off and, if possible, allow the pressure to come down naturally. If time is short, hold the pan under the cold water faucet to release the pressure. This rice has a very interesting nutty taste.

VARIATIONS WITH COOKED RICE

Just before you set the rice to cook, whichever method you choose, you can add a handful of sesame seeds (a good source of calcium) or pine nuts or sunflower seeds to give some variety.

CURRIED RICE

Serves 4

This is a good recipe for using up leftover brown rice, or you can cook fresh rice if you have none available.

1 tablespoon olive oil or 2 tablespoons (25g.) butter
1 onion, chopped
1 teaspoon mild curry powder
¼ cup (50g.) raisins
½ cup (50g.) blanched almonds, finely chopped
1½ cups (230g.) cooked long-grain brown rice

Heat the oil or butter in a frying pan or large saucepan, and fry the onion for 4–5 minutes until soft.

Add the curry powder and cook, stirring, for 1 minute. Add the raisins and almonds and stir well. Add the rice and combine well.

Cook over a low heat, stirring, for 1–2 minutes or until the rice is warm.

SHEPHERDESS PIE

Serves 4

This variation on a traditional English meat dish, shepherd's pie, is an excellent dish for serving up lentils to those who don't normally eat them. Seaweed is also used in this recipe, but in such a way that you can't taste it, yet you get all the valuable trace ingredients, so it is a very easy way of introducing it into the diet. I usually cook a double quantity of the base for this pie and freeze half. Frozen meals aren't ideal, but this way at least I know what's gone into the dish and I can add the potato topping on the day that I serve it.

¾ cup (175g.) brown lentils
2in. (5cm.) piece kombu seaweed
1 medium onion, sliced
1 garlic clove, crushed

1¾ cup (400g.) canned tomatoes
Pinch of mixed herbs
1 teaspoon soy sauce (or to taste)
1 teaspoon miso (or to taste)
1 tablespoon Westbrae Natural ketchup
1 tablespoon olive oil

For the potato topping:
2 lbs. (100g.) potatoes, organic if possible
Pinch of sea salt
Drizzle of soy milk
1 tablespoon unhydrogenated margarine or butter

In a pressure cooker or heavy saucepan with a lid, put the brown lentils together with the piece of kombu and enough water to cover. Cook until the lentils are soft, adding more water if necessary.

For the topping, put the potatoes into another pan, cover with water, add salt, and bring to the boil. Simmer until just soft. Then drain and mash with the soy milk and margarine or butter.

In the meantime, lightly sauté the sliced onion with the garlic in the olive oil in a large frying pan or wok (you need a pan with slightly higher sides than a regular frying pan) until they are soft. Add the tomatoes and mixed herbs.

When the lentils are cooked, drain them, saving any excess cooking water, and add them to the tomato mixture. Keeping the heat low, stir well. Add the soy sauce, miso, and ketchup. As you get used to cooking this dish, you can alter these last ingredients to suit your taste. Simmer for 5 minutes more.

Put the lentil mixture in a blender for just a short while with a little of the reserved lentil cooking water. This mixture forms the base of the pie, so it needs to be firm and not too runny.

Put the lentil mixture in a casserole dish with the mashed potato topping, and place in a preheated oven at 180°C (350°F) until the mashed potato is slightly brown.

If you wish, you can sprinkle a little grated cheese on top of the potato just before it goes into the oven.

VEGETABLE AND CHEESE BATTER PUDDING

Serves 6

For this recipe many different vegetables can be used, but hard vegetables such as butternut squash or rutabagas will need to be pre-cooked a little. This can be done by roasting them in the oven with a little extra-virgin olive oil and adding the batter when they are partially cooked.

4 free-range eggs
2 cups (225g.) whole-wheat flour
8½fl.oz. (250ml.) soy milk
1 tablespoon fresh parsley, chopped
1 tablespoon fresh thyme, chopped
1 tablespoon fresh tarragon, chopped
Pepper to taste
3 tablespoons extra-virgin olive oil
6 mushrooms (try shiitake mushrooms), halved
1 leek, sliced
6 baby tomatoes
8 broccoli florets
½ each of green, yellow, red, and orange bell pepper, sliced,
1½ cups (225g.) Cheddar cheese, cut into cubes

Preheat the oven to 400°F (200°C).

Make the batter by beating the eggs into the sieved flour and gradually adding the soy milk. Beat well with a wooden spoon until no lumps remain. Add the chopped herbs and pepper, and leave the batter to rest while you prepare the other vegetables.

Heat the oil in a baking dish in the oven until hot. Add the batter, then the vegetables and cheese. Bake for about 20–30 minutes until well risen and golden.

Serve with vegetable gravy and fresh salad.

SOYBEAN CASSEROLE

Serves 4

If using dried soybeans, be sure to soak overnight. Boil rapidly for 1 hour and simmer for another hour or pressure-cook for about 30 minutes. Canned beans can be used: rinse well if you have to buy beans with salt added. Fresh vegetable stock, salt- and additive-free, is available in some supermarkets.

1 teaspoon extra-virgin olive oil
1 teaspoon grated fresh root ginger
2 garlic cloves, crushed
½ teaspoon chili powder
6 green onions
4 cups (350g.) mushrooms
4 stalks celery, without leaves, cut into strips
2 carrots, cut into strips
¾ cup (90g.) water chestnuts, thinly sliced
3 tablespoons (20g.) cornstarch
1 teaspoon red wine (optional)
1 tablespoon soy sauce
1¼ cup (300ml.) water or vegetable stock
½ cup (100g.) cooked soybeans
Freshly ground black pepper

Heat the oil in a large saucepan, and sauté the ginger and garlic with the chili powder for 2–3 minutes.

Add the vegetables, including the water chestnuts, and continue cooking for 10 minutes over gentle heat with the lid on.

Mix the cornstarch, red wine, and soy sauce in a bowl and stir in the water or vegetable stock. Add this to the vegetable, together with the cooked soybeans. Stir, bring to the boil, cover, and simmer for 10 minutes.

Season with black pepper to taste before serving.

VEGETABLE AND LENTIL CURRY (THAI STYLE)

Serves 4

This recipe is great for using up leftover vegetables. Most vegetables can be used, but I list the tried and trusted. You can omit the lentils if you wish and make a less substantial meal. Go easy on the coconut milk, though, as this contains saturated fats, but it's OK in small amounts. Accompany with plain rice: a basmati is good. My family enjoys this dish with Mexican tortillas, but check the ingredients on the package if buying readymade.

1 large onion, sliced
8 mushrooms, sliced
3 garlic cloves
2 tablespoons chopped lemon grass
1 cup (300ml.) vegetable stock
1¾ cup (400g.) canned tomatoes
1 large sweet potato, peeled and cut into cubes
1 large potato, peeled and cut into cubes
8 baby squash (patty pan, if available), quartered
1 zucchini, thickly sliced
2 parsnips, peeled and sliced
2 carrots, scraped and sliced
1 eggplant chopped
2 cups (450g.) brown lentils (no need to pre-soak)
⅝ cup (100g.) sieved tomatoes
2 teaspoons chopped fresh coriander
1 teaspoon grated lime rind
1 teaspoon turmeric
½ teaspoon cumin seeds
2 teaspoons Thai green curry paste
1 large unpeeled apple, chopped
1 banana
1¼ cup (300ml.) coconut milk

Cook the onion, mushrooms, garlic, and lemon grass a little in a non-stick pan with a small amount of the stock. Add the tomatoes and the rest of the vegetables and the remaining vegetable stock. Cook for a couple of minutes.

Add the lentils, sieved tomatoes, coriander, lime rind, and spices. Cook for 15 minutes. Finally, add the apple, banana, and coconut milk. Add a little more of the spices and coconut milk according to taste, if desired. Cook over low heat for approximately 30 minutes until the vegetables are very soft.

PASTA WITH LENTILS AND SPINACH

Serves 4

1 cup (230g.) uncooked red lentils
1 lb. (450g.) dried whole-wheat spaghetti
1 onion, finely chopped
1 teaspoon grated nutmeg
1 teaspoon extra-virgin olive oil
10 spinach leaves, shredded
1 tablespoon lemon juice
½ cup (50g.) toasted pine nuts
Lemon quarters, to serve

Cook the lentils in boiling water until tender, then drain.
Cook the pasta separately in unsalted boiling water until
just tender, then drain. Meanwhile fry the onion and nutmeg
in the olive oil until the onion is soft. Add the spinach and
cook, covered, until it is tender.

Add lemon juice, drained lentils, and the cooked pasta.
Serve sprinkled with the pine nuts and accompanied by the
lemon quarters for squeezing.

Spinach contains high amounts of oxalic acid, which has
been implicated in kidney-stone formation, so use it sparingly.

HAZELNUT AND ZUCCHINI ROAST

Serves 4

1 medium onion, chopped
3 tablespoons sunflower or safflower oil
¾ cup (100g.) hazelnuts, chopped
1¼ lb. (500g.) zucchini, diced
½ tablespoon sesame seeds
½ tablespoon cumin seeds
½ teaspoon turmeric
1 tablespoon fresh root ginger, chopped
¾ cup (75g.) organic rolled oats

¾ cup (75g.) ground nuts (peanuts, cashews, or almonds)
⅝ cup (50g.) creamed coconut, grated
Pinch of freshly ground black pepper
1 cup (150g.) sieved tomatoes

Preheat the oven to 350°F (180°C). Sauté the onions in half the oil until soft. Add the hazelnuts and zucchini, and cook for 10 minutes until the zucchini are soft. Heat the rest of the oil, and cook the sesame seeds, cumin, turmeric, and ginger for 2–3 minutes. Combine this mixture with the onions and hazelnuts and add the oats, ground nuts, coconut, and pepper. Stir in the sieved tomatoes. Grease a small bread pan (approx. 6 ½ × 4 ½ × 3in. [17 × 11 × 7cm.]), and press the mixture into it. Bake for 35 minutes.

BOUILLABAISSE

Serves 4–6

2 tablespoons olive oil
1 large onion, sliced
2 garlic cloves, crushed
3½ cups (400g.) canned chopped tomatoes
1¼ pint (600ml.) fish or vegetable stock
Sea salt and freshly ground pepper to taste
1–2 drops soy sauce
1 bouquet garni
1 large bay leaf
Pinch of saffron strands
1½–2lbs. (675–900g.) mixed fish fillets (monkfish, cod, haddock), skinned and cubed
6–7oz. (175–200g.) peeled shrimp
Chopped fresh parsley to garnish

Heat the oil and sauté the onion and garlic until soft. Stir in the tomatoes, stock, seasoning, soy sauce, bouquet garni, bay leaf, and saffron. Bring to the boil and simmer for 10 minutes.

Add the cubes of fish and simmer for 2–3 minutes. Stir in shrimp and cook for 2 minutes.

Remove the bouquet garni and the bay leaf. Sprinkle with parsley and serve with a fresh mixed salad.

FISH AND TOMATO HOT POT

Serves 4

1 tablespoon olive oil
1 medium onion, sliced
1 eggplant cubed
½ cup (100g.) green beans, chopped
6 small fresh tomatoes, skinned, de-seeded, and
chopped or 1¾ cup (400g.) canned tomatoes
3 tablespoons tomato paste
Sea salt and freshly ground black pepper to taste
1lb. (450g.) fillet of cod, or other firm, white fish, cut into
cubes
1lb. (450g.) new potatoes, scrubbed, sliced, and cooked
1 tablespoon chopped fresh parsley, to garnish

Heat the oil in a large, shallow pan. Add the sliced onion and cook until soft and translucent. Add the eggplant cubes and cook for 1 minute. Add the beans, tomatoes, tomato paste, seasoning, and 5 tablespoons of water. Simmer, uncovered, for 5 minutes. Add the fish and potatoes. Stir, then cook, uncovered, for 5–7 minutes until the fish is just cooked through. Garnish with the chopped parsley and serve immediately.

BROILED SALMON STEAKS WITH TERIYAKI SAUCE

Serves 4

In this dish a classic Japanese teriyaki sauce is used as a glaze. Once made, it can be stored in a jar in the refrigerator for a long time. The two more unusual Japanese ingredients, sake and mirin, give a wonderful flavor to food, and since they both last indefinitely, would be worthwhile keeping in the kitchen. Sake is Japanese rice wine, and mirin is Japanese sweet white rice wine. You can have this dish as a special treat, though it is quick enough to cook at the end of a working day.

4 salmon steaks, approximately 1in. (2.5cm.) thick

For the teriyaki sauce:
⅓ cup (75 ml.) sake
⅓ cup (75 ml.) mirin
⅓ cup (75 ml.) soy sauce
2 teaspoons clear honey or maple syrup

To make the sauce, mix all the sauce ingredients together in a small saucepan and bring to the boil over a medium heat. Cook until the honey is dissolved.

Broil the salmon for about 3–5 minutes on one side. Baste with the sauce, turn, baste again, and continue to cook for 3–5 minutes more.

TOFU

Tofu is soybean curd, made from yellow soybeans. By itself it has no taste: its flavor is dependent on what you cook with it. It is very versatile because of this ability to pick up the taste of whatever you combine it with and because it can be prepared in a variety of ways. It can be sliced, cubed, mashed, scrambled, puréed and used in savory and sweet dishes. So you can find tofu in soups, stir-fries, baked in casserole, in dips, dressings, sauces, and desserts.

Add tofu to an ordinary stir-fry simply by cutting it into cubes and cooking it with the other ingredients. Add strong flavors, such as garlic, ginger, tamari, etc., which the tofu will absorb.

My family prefers a very simple way of eating tofu. I cut it into thin slices rather than cubes, and lightly fry it in olive oil. At the end of cooking, when it is pale brown and the pan is still hot, I sprinkle the tofu with tamari and gently turn it over. It is eaten as it is, often simply with brown rice and vegetables, or used in sandwiches with mayonnaise, mustard, and lettuce.

FRIED SESAME TOFU

This dish is fried, which is not a means of cooking to be recommended regularly, but if you are using tofu as a beginner, it does make a delicious dish.

5 tablespoons sesame seeds
1lb. (450g.) tofu
5 tablespoons fine milled whole-wheat flour
2 free-range eggs, beaten
6 tablespoons sesame oil

For the dipping sauce:
4 tablespoons mirin
4 tablespoons brown rice vinegar
¼ cup (60ml.) tamari
2 teaspoons maple syrup

First roast the sesame seeds. This can done in two ways, either by spreading on a baking sheet and placing in a preheated oven at 160°C (325°F) until they are slightly brown or by dry roasting in a frying pan. With the latter method they need to be stirred continuously, so that they brown evenly. You can tell they are done by taking a pinch of the seeds and rubbing them between your finger and thumb: if they split and crack, they are ready to use.

Empty the water from the tofu pack, and dry the tofu with paper towels. Cube the tofu into 1in. (2.5cm.) pieces. Toss the tofu in the flour, then dip in the beaten eggs and sprinkle on the sesame seeds.

Use a deep frying pan or wok to heat the oil to a medium heat, and then add the tofu cubes. Let the tofu brown gently on both sides, turning as necessary. Drain off excess oil by placing the tofu cubes on paper towels. Since you will have to do this in several batches, place the cooked tofu in a very low oven to keep it warm while the next batch is cooking.

To make the sauce, mix all the ingredients together; serve with the tofu.

TOFU PILAF

Serves 4

1⅓ cups (350g.) long-grain brown rice
1 tablespoon olive oil
2 medium onions, chopped
2 bay leaves
Pinch of sea salt
2 teaspoons turmeric
2 teaspoons garam masala
2 teaspoons lemon juice
1 package (approx. 10oz. [285g.]) of tofu, cubed

Wash the rice and drain well. Heat half the oil, and sauté the onions for 3–4 minutes. Add the rice, bay leaves, and sea salt, cover with boiling water, and simmer until the rice is almost tender. Add the remainder of the oil to another pan, add the turmeric and garam masala, and cook for 3–4 minutes, then add the lemon juice. Stir in the tofu, and leave to cook gently for 3–4 minutes. About 5 minutes before the rice is ready, add the tofu mixture and stir well. Continue simmering until the rice is tender and the water is absorbed. Before serving, remove the bay leaves.

SEAWEED

Nori is the seaweed used by the Japanese to make a form of sushi (nori wrapped around rice with cucumber or fish in the middle). It is usually bought in sheets and toasted in the oven, where it changes from brown to green. It can then be crumbled and used as a condiment to put on rice or pasta or added to soups. My family eats it cut up in squares; it is quite crisp once toasted.

Kombu, the Japanese equivalent of kelp, is very helpful for avoiding the flatulence that can be caused by beans. Just cut off about 2in. (5cm.)—kombu comes in flat strips—and after discarding the soaking water from the beans, use the kombu in the cooking water. At the end of cooking, the kombu will be quite soft and you can break it up and eat it with the beans or remove it. Kombu helps to break down the starch molecules in beans which cause flatulence, and you will get the goodness from the kombu itself, too.

Sauces

SWEET-AND-SOUR SAUCE

This is an easy-to-make sauce, and yet it can change a very simple meal. You can use it poured over plain brown rice or mixed in at the end of a tofu and vegetable stir-fry or just to brighten up some leftover vegetables.

> 2 tablespoons arrowroot
> 2 tablespoons water
> 1 cup (235ml.) unsweetened apple juice
> ⅓ cup (80ml.) cider vinegar
> ¼ cup (60ml.) honey or maple syrup
> 1 tablespoon soy sauce

Put the arrowroot and water together in a small bowl, and mix to a smooth paste.

Place the other ingredients in a small saucepan, and heat over a medium flame. Gradually add the arrowroot paste to the apple juice mix until you get the consistency of sauce that you prefer. Serve hot.

MARINADE FOR FISH

It is worthwhile leaving fish for a couple of hours in a marinade. Try this one for fresh tuna fish. Baste the fish with the marinade while broiling.

> ½ cup (120ml.) extra-virgin olive oil
> 1 tablespoon fresh root ginger, grated

Juice and grated rind of 1 lime
2 tablespoons balsamic vinegar

Simply mix together all the ingredients.

Tarragon and Dill Sauce

This sauce is delicious with salmon, though it goes well with most other fish, too. Broil the fish first, lightly brushing with oil. Or gently pan fry in a frying pan, using a touch of oil. The fish can also be cut into thin strips and cooked, but be careful not to overcook—only 2 minutes per side is needed.

1¼ (600ml.) pints fish stock (can be bought from some
supermarkets)
¾ cup (175ml.) heavy cream or thick soy "cream"
Juice of 1 lemon
2 tablespoons fresh tarragon, chopped
1 tablespoon fresh dill, chopped

Simmer the fish stock and half the cream in a pan until reduced by half. Add the rest of the cream and the lemon juice, and reduce a little more. Add most of the chopped tarragon and dill. Simply pour over the cooked fish of your choice and sprinkle with the reserved herbs.

Salads

Rice Salad

This salad can be made a day ahead for convenience.

1 cup (200g.) mixed wild and basmati brown or white rice
6 green onions, chopped
½ cucumber, chopped
2 red peppers, chopped
1 yellow pepper, chopped
½ cup (20g.) chopped fresh parsley

For the dressing:
2 teaspoons concentrated apple juice
3 teaspoons curry powder
1¼ cups (300ml.) sunflower or safflower oil
1½ tablespoons cider vinegar

Rinse the rice, then boil in unsalted water for 20–30 minutes. Drain and allow to cool. Add the vegetables and parsley. Combine all the dressing ingredients, and pour over the salad just before serving.

GENERAL-PURPOSE SALAD DRESSING I

This dressing goes superbly with any salad. Keep some in the fridge to use on salads at any time. Walnut oil (studies have shown it is good for the heart) gives a lovely nutty flavor, and the vinegar complements this. Dress up a little with fresh herbs such as thyme, oregano, mint, or basil.

1 cup (235ml.) walnut oil
½ cup (120ml.) champagne vinegar or white wine vinegar
Grated rind of 1 lemon

Simply mix all the ingredients together.

GENERAL-PURPOSE SALAD DRESSING II

This dressing goes well with a vegetable salad that also contains fruit such as melons, grapes, etc.

1 cup (235ml.) walnut oil
4 whole strawberries, blended
¼ cup (60ml.) strawberry vinegar or other berry vinegar
Grated rind of 1 lemon

Whisk all the ingredients together with a fork.

EDIBLE FLOWERS

In salads, try edible flowers, as they add interest, color, and valuable nutrients. You must be absolutely certain that they have not been sprayed. The best way is to grow them in the garden along with some common herbs. They can be grown in pots outside your back door to be cut as needed. Try nasturtiums, pansies (in warm climates you can grow these in winter), marigolds, violas, and rose petals. Make sure the flowers are edible, though: if in doubt, don't use. Herbs such as various mints, oregano, parsley, thyme, chives, and rosemary are easy to grow. You can use the flowers of these herbs for salads.

Try any of these flowers with green and red salad leaves such as Boston lettuce, corn salad, sorrel, and baby spinach. Drizzle in one of the above dressings, and enjoy.

VEGETABLE JULIENNE SALAD

Serves 4

The prepared vegetables will keep in the fridge for a day, covered. But once dressing is added, this salad is best eaten as soon as possible.

2 carrots, cut into thin julienne (matchstick) strips
2 celery stalks cut into julienne strips
1 red, 1 yellow, 1 orange, and 1 green pepper, cut into julienne strips
1 teaspoon clear honey or maple syrup
1 tablespoon fresh mint, chopped

For the dressing:
1 teaspoon fresh mint, chopped
2 tablespoons hazelnut oil
1 tablespoon champagne vinegar or wine vinegar
1 teaspoon wholegrain mustard

Mix together all the salad ingredients. Whisk together the dressing ingredients. Toss the salad with the dressing.

BEET SALAD

3 whole fresh beets, peeled and grated
2 large carrots, peeled and grated

For the dressing:
½ cup (120ml.) orange juice
2 teaspoons grated orange rind
1 tablespoon tahini
½ small red chili, finely chopped
1 tablespoon sesame seeds, toasted

Combine the grated beet and carrot. Separately combine the orange juice and rind, tahini, chili, and sesame seeds, whisking well. Pour this dressing over the vegetables.

Desserts and cakes

Now you might be thinking that although main and first courses seem quite straightforward, if sugar is not so good for you, what are you going to do for desserts? You are not going to be deprived, but you will rarely be able to buy ready made desserts at the supermarket.

This part of the meal, I feel, requires more effort, but desserts can be very simple. Obviously fresh fruit compotes, baked apples stuffed with nuts and raisins, and live yogurt are all easy options. I often adapt recipes for ordinary desserts just by altering a few ingredients, and this usually works out extremely well.

JELLIED DESSERTS

Gelatin-type desserts can be made with agar, an easy introduction to seaweeds. Agar Agar Seaweed Gel, by Eden Foods, is available from health food stores and comes in flake form. You may also find agar in the form of a powder or a bar. Instructions for use vary from one product to another. For a delicious and colorful dessert, combine the agar with boiled fruit juice, such as grape or cranberry juice, and, as it sets, add chopped or sliced fruit, such as halves of seedless grapes or segments of mandarin oranges (canned in fruit juice, not syrup).

BAKED BANANAS

This is a quick and easy dessert. You can vary it by using orange juice instead of lemon and sprinkling with ground cloves and cinnamon.

4 bananas, peeled and sliced lengthwise
4 tablespoons lemon juice
4 tablespoons clear honey or maple syrup
4 tablespoons dried or fresh shredded coconut

Preheat the oven to 180°C (350°F). Place the bananas in a baking dish. Cover with the lemon juice and honey or maple syrup. Sprinkle on the coconut. Cover with a lid, and bake for 15–20 minutes.

TOFU FRUIT WHIP

Serve this topped with slices of fresh fruit, your favorite breakfast cereal or Crunchy Oat Cereal (page 228).

4 oz. (100g.)—approx. ⅝ cup—tofu, drained
1 cup (100mg.) fresh fruit, (strawberries, pears, peaches, black currants, etc.)
Maple syrup to taste
Dash of vanilla extract
1 tablespoon tahini (optional)

Blend all the ingredients until smooth. For a creamier taste, you can add a spoonful of tahini.

CARROT AND RAISIN LOAF

For this recipe, measure out the flour first in a measuring cup, then the oil, and then the honey. By doing the oil before the honey, you prevent the honey from sticking to the cup.

½ cup (125ml.) sunflower oil
⅜ cup (100ml.) clear honey
2 eggs
2⅔ cup (225g.) carrots, grated
¾ cup (100g.) raisins
½ teaspoon baking powder
1⅞ cups (200g.) whole-wheat flour
½ teaspoon ground cinnamon
¼ teaspoon grated nutmeg
¼ teaspoon ground mixed spice

Preheat the oven to 325°F (170°C). Grease a small bread pan.

Beat the oil, honey, and eggs together until smooth. Add the carrots and raisins, and combine gently. Fold in the baking powder, flour, and spices. Spoon into the pan and bake for 1¼ hours. Leave to cool, then remove from the pan.

DATE SLICE

This is delicious and sweet, yet contains no added sugar. It freezes well—but doesn't get much chance to get into the freezer in my house.

3 cups (700g.) dates, stoned and roughly chopped
4½ cups (450g.) rolled oats
2 cups (225g.) whole-wheat flour
¾ cup (175ml.) barley malt syrup
¾ cup (175ml.) sunflower oil

Preheat the oven to 350°F (180°C). Grease a 10 × 12in. (25 × 30cm.) baking pan or dish.

Place the dates in a saucepan and cover with water. Simmer until the dates are soft.

Combine the oats and flour in blender. Add the malt and oil, and blend thoroughly.

Put three-quarters of the oat mixture in the bottom of the greased pan, and press it down well with your hands. Spread the dates over the top. Spread the remaining oat mixture on top of the dates. Bake for 40 minutes or until brown.

OAT BARS

These are a family favorite and are easy to make. The use of barley malt syrup instead of another sweetener like honey makes them very tasty.

½ cup (100g.) unhydrogenated margarine
½ cup (150g.) barley malt syrup
2⅛ cups (225g.) rolled oats (organic if possible)

Preheat the oven to 325°F (165°C). In a saucepan, melt the margarine and barley malt together gently so that they do not burn. Put the oats in a large bowl, and then add the melted margarine/malt mixture and combine thoroughly. Grease a rectangular cake pan, and press the mixture into the bottom so that it is approximately ½–1 in. (1–2.5cm.) thick. I actually prefer thinner, crispier bars and spread out the mixture accordingly. Bake in the oven for 25 minutes.

The end? No, just the beginning

I feel strongly that our first choice should always be the natural approach—i.e., natural diet, natural lifestyle, natural nutritional supplements, and exercise, because the menopause is a natural event in your life. The alternative is HRT, which should be kept as our last resort.

You are now at the crossroads of a new beginning: achieving good health and a positive future is in your hands. If you need advice from a health professional, don't be intimidated by the first person you see: get a second or third opinion. Gather all the information you can find and look for a doctor with whom you feel comfortable and can discuss the different approaches that may meet your individual needs. In this book I have outlined the choices available to you and explained the options. It is your body and your choice. You can now use this information to ask the right questions, understand the answers, and then make up your own mind as to what treatment or direction you want to take for the rest of your life. With this knowledge you can take control of your health and go forward with confidence into the next phase of your life.

References

CHAPTER 3
What is Hormone Replacement Therapy (HRT)?

1. R. Hoover et al., *New England Journal of Medicine* (1976), 295, 401–5
2. H. Ziel and W. Finkle, *New England Journal of Medicine* (1975), 293, 1167–70
3. Smith et al., *New England Journal of Medicine* (1975), 293, 1164–67
4. *Annals of Inter Medicine* (1992), 1777. 12. 1016–37
5. *British Medical Journal*, February 17, 1990
6. *Obstetrics and Gynaecology*, February 1992
7. M. D. Bergavist et al., *New England Journal of Medicine* (1989), 321, 5, 293–8
8. Ibid.
9. I. Persson et al., *The Lancet* (1992), 340, 1044
10. P. W. F. Wilson, R. J. Garison, W. P. Castelli, *New England Journal of Medicine* (1985), 513, 1038–43
11. D. T. Felson et al., *New England Journal of Medicine* (1993), 329, 1141–6
12. F. Pollner, *Medical World News* (1985), January 14, 38–58

CHAPTER 4
"Natural" progesterone—why this is not the answer either

1. J. Lee, *What Your Doctor May Not Tell You About the Menopause* (1996)
2. Mauvis-Jarvis et al., *Pecutaneous Absorption of Steroids* (1980)
3. D. Grimes, *Fertility and Sterility*, (1992), 57, 3, 492–3
4. International Agency for Research on Cancer (IARC), "Monographs on the Evaluation of the Carcinogenic risk of Chemicals to Humans," December 1979

CHAPTER 5
Best nutrition for the menopause

1. H. Adlercreutz, *The Lancet* (1992), 339-1233
   J. W. Erdman, *New England Journal of Medicine* (1995), 333, 313-315
   J. Ziegler, *Journal of the National Cancer Institute* (1994), 86, 1666-7

CHAPTER 6
Natural alternatives to HRT

1. F. Wilcox et al., *British Medical Journal* (1993), 301, 905–906
2. Mursa et al., *Asia Oceania Journal of Obstetrics and Gynaecology* (1984), 10, 3, 317
3. 9th Int. Congress in Prosta, Florence, 1994
4. J. P. Minton et al., *Surgery* (1979), 86, 105–9
5. D. J. Ingram, *Journal of the National Cancer Institute* (1987), 79, 1225
   D. Rose, *Journal of the National Cancer Institute* (1987), 78, 623
   W. Willet et al., *New England Journal of Medicine* (1987), 316, 22
6. J. Hargrave and G. Abraham, *Infertility* (1979), 2:315
7. N. L. Petrakis and E. B. King, *The Lancet* (1981), ii, 1, 203–5
8. H. Hikon et al., *Planta Medica* (1984), 50, 248–50
   G. Vogel et al., *Arzneim-Forsch* (1975), 25, 179–85
   H. Wagner in J. L. Beal and E. Reinhard (eds.), *Natural Products as Medicinal Agents* (1981)
9. E. J. Johnson et al., *British Medical Journal*, (1985), 291, 569–73
10. D. Lithgow and W. Politzer, *South African Medical Journal* (1977), 51, 191–3
11. J. D. Cohen and H. W. Rubin, *Current Therapeutic Research* (1960), 2, 539–42
12. C. J. Smith, *Chicago Medicine* (1964), March 7
13. C. J. Christy, *American Journal of Obstetrics* (1945), 50–84
    B. B. Rubenstein, *Federation Proceedings* (Federation of American Societies for Experimental Biology) (1948), 7, 106
    R. S. Finkler, *Journal of Clinical Endocrinology and Metabolism* (1949), 9, 89–94
14. E. J. Shute, *Journal of Obstetrics and Gynaecology of the British Empire* (1942), 49, 482
15. E. Racz-Kotilla et al., *Planta Medica* (1974), 26, 212–17

CHAPTER 7
What is osteoporosis?

1. C. D. P. Wright et al., *British Medical Journal* (1993), 306, 429–30
2. B. T. Lees et al., *The Lancet* (1993), 341, 673–75
3. *American Journal of Clinical Nutrition* (1988)
4. Kronre et al., *Clinical Science* (1983), 64, 541–6
   R. Yeater and R. Martin, *Postgraduate Medicine* (1984), 75, 147–9
5. T. L. Holbrook and E. Barrett-Conner, *British Medical Journal* (1993), 1056–8
   S. S. Harris and B. Dawson-Hughest, *American Journal of Clinical Nutrition* (1994), 60, 573–9
6. L. Rose, *Osteoporosis* (1994)
7. K. Kin et al., *Calcification Tissue International* (1991), 49, 101–6
8. A. Wynn and M. Wynn, *Journal of Nutritional and Environmental Medicine* (1995), 5, 41–53
9. C. Cooper et al., *British Medical Journal* (1988), 297, 1443–6
10. N. Kreiger et al., *American Journal of Epidemiology* (1982), 116, 141, 8
11. *Alternative Medicine* (1994)
12. J. N. Hunt and C. Johnson, *Digestive Diseases and Sciences* (1983), 28, 5, 417–21
13. J. A. Harvey et al., *Journal of Bone Mineral Research* (1988), 3, 3, 253–8
14. *Current Research in Osteoporosis and Bone Mineral Measurement*, II, British Institute of Radiology (1992)
15. G. E. Abraham, *Journal of Nutritional Medicine* (1991), 2, 165–78
16. A. Gaby and J. Wright, "Nutrients and Bone Health," *Green Farm Magazine*, spring 1994
17. R Nuti, et al., *Osteoporosis International* (1993), 3, 59–65

CHAPTER 8
Your breasts at the menopause

1. M. P. Coleman et al., *Trends in Cancer Incidence and Mortality* (1993) Lyon, France, IARC Publication, no. 121
2. Presented at the European Society for Therapeutic Radiology and Oncology, 1996
3. *Journal of Nutrition* (1995), 125, 437–445
4. K. K. Steinberg et al., *Epidemiology* (1994), 5, 415–21
5. L. Bernstein, *Journal of the National Cancer Institute* (1994), 86, 18
6. D. L. Davis et al., *Environmental Health Perspectives* (October 1993), 1001, 5, 377–8

7. *Canadian Journal of Public Health* (1993), 84, 14–16
8. R. Singer and S. Grismaijer, *Dressed to Kill—The Link Between Breast Cancer and Bras* (Avery)
9. *Alternative Medicine—The Definitive Guide* (1994), compiled by the Burton Goldberg Group
10. A. Trichopoulous et al., *Journal of the National Cancer Institute* (1995), 87, 2, 110–16
11. J. Ziegler, "Soybeans show promise in cancer prevention," *Journal of the National Cancer Institute* (1994), 86, 1666–7
12. J. W. Erdmann, *New England Journal of Medicine* (1995), 333, 313–15
13. H. Aldercreutz et al., *The Lancet* (1992), 339, 1233
14. F. Wilcox et al., *British Medical Journal* (1993), 301, 905–6

Chapter 9
Your heart at the menopause

1. *Journal of the American Medical Association* (August 1996)
2. Coronary Drug Project Research Group (1973), *Journal of the American Medicine Association*, 226, 652–57
3. M. J. Stampfer et al., *New England Journal of Medicine* (1985), 313, 1044–9
4. P. W. F. Wilson et al., *New England Journal of Medicine* (1985), 313, 1038–43
5. S. D. Grodstein et al., *New England Journal of Medicine* (1996), 335, 7, 453–61
6. J. C. Prior, Letter in *New England Journal of Medicine* (1992), 326, 705–6
7. E. Barrett-Connor and D. Gooidman-Gruen, *British Medical Journal* (1995), 311, 1193–6
8. W. J. Elliot, *American Journal of Medicine* (1983), 75, 1024–32
9. L. Kinlen, *The Lancet* (1982), 946–9
10. N. G. Stephens et al., *The Lancet* (1996), 347, 781–6
11. *Journal of the Institute for Optimum Nutrition* (summer 1996), vol. 9, no. 2
12. B. M. Altura and B. T. Altura, *Magnesium* (1985), 4, 226–44
   P. D. M. V. Turlapaty and B. T. Altura, *Science* (1980), 208, 199–200

Chapter 10
How to control your weight and your mood

1. P. H. Langsjoen et al., *Drug Experimental and Clinical Research* (1985), XI, 8, 577
   T. Kamikawa et al., *American Journal of Cardiology* (1985), 56, 247

Y. Yamagami et al., *Research Communication in Chemical Pathology and Pharmacology* (1976), 14, 4, 721

E. G. Wilkinson et al., *Research Communication in Chemical and Clinical Pharmacology* (1975), 12, 1, 103

C. Kishimoto et al., *Japanese Circulation Journal* (1984), 48, 12, 1358

2. L. Van Gaal et al., *Biomedical and Clinical Aspects of Coenzyme Q* (1984), 4, 369

CHAPTER 11
The benefits of exercise and sex at the menopause

1. L. Twomey, *Patient Management* (1989), 29–34
2. B. Kolner et al., *Clinical Science* (1983), 64, 541–6

   R. Yester and R. Martin, *Postgraduate Medicine* (1984), 75, 147–9

CHAPTER 12
Tests at the menopause

1. H. Lene, *European Journal of Allergy and Clinical Immunology* (1995), 26, 50

   P. Fell, J. Brostoff and M. Pasula, "Annals of Allergy" (1988), presented at the 45th Annual Congress of the American College of Allergy and Immunology, California

   J. Hoj, *Journal of Allergy and Clinical Immunology* (1996), 1, 3, 97

   S. Baker, *American College of Environmental Medicine*, October 1994

Jargon busters

Aerobic exercise—increases oxygen consumption and helps the lungs and cardiovascular system. Aerobic exercises include jogging, brisk walking, swimming, etc.

Amino acids—the building blocks of protein. There are twenty-two known amino acids, but eight of these are classed as essential because they must be obtained from our food, as we cannot make them ourselves. The protein we eat is broken down by digestion into amino acids and then used to make other proteins.

Antioxidants—substances that stop oxidation when a substance is exposed to oxygen. Oxygen is essential for our bodies to function. Unfortunately, when oxidation takes place, this can create highly reactive chemical fragments called free radicals. These free radicals have been linked to cancer, coronary heart disease, rheumatoid arthritis, and premature aging. Environmental pollutants, smoking, and ultraviolet light can also increase production of free radicals. Antioxidants prevent this oxidation from taking place. They include beta-carotene, vitamin E, vitamin C, and selenium.

Arteriosclerosis—thickening of the arteries due to age or high blood pressure.

Atherosclerosis—disease of the arteries caused by fatty plaques deposited on the inner walls, making the arteries narrower.

Beta-carotene—the vegetable form of vitamin A. (The animal form of the vitamin is called retinol.) It is a powerful antioxidant and is found in many vegetables and fruits with an orange or green pigment such as carrots, dark leafy greens, and oranges.

Bioflavonoids—substances found in fruits such as blackberries, black currants, lemons, and plums. They help to increase the function of vitamin C. They also help to keep the connective tissues, such as the skin, healthy and strengthen capillary function and hence the circulation.

Chelation—a process by which minerals are made more absorbable. The label on a supplement container might state, for example, "Manganese (as amino acid chelate)."

Collagen—"cement" that holds cells together, the primary organic constituent of bone, cartilage, and connective tissue. As you get older there is a decrease in collagen, which can cause changes to your skin (wrinkles, prominent veins, slow wound healing, bruising easily), nails (brittleness), eyes (dryness, dark circles under the eyes), gums (bleeding, infection), hair (dullness, split ends, poor growth, hair loss) and mouth (bad breath, mouth ulcers).

Vitamin C's major function is to produce collagen. Collagen makes up 90 percent of our bone matrix.

Contraindication—any factor in your medical history that would mean that it would be unwise to take a particular medication or follow a certain line of treatment.

Diuretic—any substance that increases the volume of urine.

Endometriosis—an illness that causes the lining of the womb to grow elsewhere in the body.

Endorphins—brain chemicals that help us to feel happier, more alert, and calmer. Endorphins can give us a "natural buzz", a sense of euphoria.

Enzymes—proteins that in small amounts act as triggers to speed up the rate of biological reactions. They do not get used up themselves in the reaction.

Essential fatty acids—unsaturated fats are called essential fatty acids because they are essential for your health. These fats are a vital component of every human cell, and your body needs them to insulate your nerve cells, keep your skin and arteries supple, balance your hormones, and keep you warm. They are found in nuts, seeds, oily fish, and vegetables.

Ferritin—the form in which iron is stored in the body.

Fibroids—benign tumors that grow in the womb.

Follicle stimulating hormone (FSH)—hormone secreted from the pituitary gland in the brain that stimulates the ripening of the follicles in the ovary. This begins the process of ovulation by stimulating the ovaries to produce the estrogen hormones. At the menopause your FSH level rises dramatically as your body tries unsuccessfully to induce ovulation.

Free radicals—highly reactive chemical fragments which have been linked to cancer, coronary heart disease, rheumatoid arthritis, and premature aging. Environmental pollutants, smoking, ultraviolet light, overheating fats, and eating barbecued food can increase production of free radicals. Their damaging effect is stopped by antioxidants.

Gluten—protein found in wheat, oats, rye, and barley to which some people are allergic. Non-gluten grains include brown rice, millet, and buckwheat as well as flours and flakes made from these grains.

High density lipoprotein (HDL)—"good" cholesterol. HDL transports cholesterol away from the cells. The HDL level should be above 0.9mmol per liter of blood.

Inorganic—an inorganic mineral would not be found in any plant or animal. Because of this, our bodies have difficulty using it. An example is calcium carbonate (an inorganic mineral often marketed as a mineral supplement), which is mined from the ground.

Isoflavones—these chemicals form the bulk of soy protein. In the human gut, bacteria convert isoflavones into compounds that can have an estrogenic action, although they are not actually hormones.

iu(s)—international unit(s). A quantity of a biological

substance, such as a vitamin, that produces a particular effect, agreed upon by an international standard.

Kyphosis—an outward curving of the spine causing a hunching effect, commonly known as dowager's hump.

Luteinizing hormone (LH)—the hormone released by the pituitary gland that causes ovulation.

Lymph—fluid that bathes all the tissues. The lymphatic system plays an important part in immune function by getting rid of toxins from the body.

Mastalgia—chronic pain in the breast.

Metabolism—all the physical and chemical processes that take place in the body in order for it to grow and function.

Methylxanthine—an active ingredient in caffeine which has been linked to benign breast disease.

Neurotransmitters—brain chemicals that transmit signals to neurones (brain cells).

Opposed HRT—estrogen and progestogen are taken together as Hormone Replacement Therapy.

Organic—fruits, vegetables, and grains grown without the use of chemical fertilizers and pesticides.

Phytoestrogens—a group of foods which contain substances that have a hormone-like action. Examples are soybeans, fennel, celery, parsley, clover, and linseed oil.

Saturated fats—a fat is saturated when its molecules hold the maximum amount of hydrogen. The more saturated a fat becomes, the harder it is for your body to use it, and so the fat gets deposited and stored. Saturated fats include hard cheese, butter, and palm oil.

Steroids—compounds with a particular chemical structure and including the naturally occurring hormones: estrogens, progesterone, and testosterone.

Tincture—a liquid way of taking herbs which is a mixture of water and alcohol. The alcohol acts as a preservative.

Trans fatty acids—the process of hydrogenation in food

manufacturing changes the essential unsaturated fats contained in food into trans fatty acids. These have been linked to an increased rate of heart attack.

Unopposed HRT—Hormone Replacement Therapy given as estrogen only: no progestogen is added into the regime.

Unsaturated fats—fats that are usually liquid at room temperature, such as vegetable oils. They are essential for health and hence are classed as essential fatty acids.

Suggested further reading

Books on the menopause

Coney, Sandra, *The Menopause Industry* (Penguin Books, 1991)

Grant, Ellen, *Sexual Chemistry* (Cedar, 1994)

Greer, Germaine, *The Change* (Penguin, 1991)

Northrup, Christine, *Women's Bodies, Women's Wisdom* (Piatkus, 1995)

Sheehy, Gail, *The Silent Passage* (HarperCollins, 1991)

Food and cooking

Cousins, Barbara, *Cooking Without* (Barbara Cousins, 1989), a useful book if you want to eliminate certain foods from your diet for a while, such as wheat, sugar, eggs and dairy products

Lebrecht, Elbie, *Sugar Free Cooking* (Thorsons, 1994)

Marsden, Kathryn, *The Food Combining Diet* (Thorsons, 1993)

Any cookery books by Sara Brown and Delia Smith. Delia Smith uses good quantities of 'clean', fresh ingredients.

General health

Budd, Martin, *Low Blood Sugar* (Thorsons, 1984)

Lazarides, Linda, *The Principles of Nutritional Therapy* (Thorsons, 1995)

What Doctors Don't Tell You, a well-researched monthly publication. Subscription department: 4 Wallace Road, London N1 2PG.

Index

About the author

Dr. Marilyn Glenville obtained her doctorate from Cambridge University, England, and is a chartered psychologist. For over twenty years she has studied and practiced Nutritional Medicine, both in Britain and in the United States, specializing in the natural approach to female hormone problems. She has had several papers published in scientific journals, is a frequent speaker on BBC radio, and has often appeared on British television and in the British press. Dr. Glenville regularly conducts seminars and workshops throughout Britain, and she is a popular international speaker. She runs four private clinics in London, Kent, and Sussex.